Heredity and Ability

How Genetics Affects
Your Child and
What You Can Do About It

Heredity and Ability

How Genetics Affects Your Child and What You Can Do About It

Charles M. Strom, M.D., Ph.D.

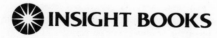 **INSIGHT BOOKS**

Plenum Press • New York and London

Library of Congress Cataloging-in-Publication Data

Strom, Charles.
   Heredity and ability : how genetics affects your child and what
you can do about it / Charles M. Strom.
      p.   cm.
   Includes bibliographical references and index.
   ISBN 0-306-43560-8
   1. Mental retardation--Etiology.   2. Mental retardation--Genetic
aspects.   3. Human chromosome abnormalities--Diagnosis.
4. Mentallly handicapped children.   I. Title.
RJ506.M4S76   1990
618.92'8588--dc20   90-39720
                                                                CIP

ISBN 0-306-43560-8

© 1990 Charles M. Strom
Plenum Press is a Division of
Plenum Publishing Corporation
233 Spring Street, New York, N.Y. 10013

An Insight Book

Printed in the United States of America

Preface

I am a geneticist practicing in the Chicago area. One of my special interests is the diagnosis and treatment of children with birth defects, genetic diseases, mental retardation, learning disabilities, and behavior disorders.

In the spring of 1987, I was fortunate enough to be given a tour of the Laremont School. Laremont provides educational services for handicapped children in the Special Education District of Lake County, Illinois. My tour was arranged by Dr. Jay Hirsch, a good friend and colleague who specializes in child and adolescent psychiatry and was a medical advisor to the Special Education District of Lake County at the time of my visit. My morning at that facility had a profound impact on me.

I was tremendously impressed by the entire staff, not just for their dedication and effort in working with these children, but for their obvious affection for their students. Everyone, from the teachers and teachers' aides to the school nurse and the administrative staff, knew most of the students by name and was intimately familiar with their strengths, weaknesses, and special problems. During my visit to Laremont the staff bombarded me with medical and genetic questions about individual students and about general pediatric and medical issues regarding the diagnosis and care of handicapped children. I was amazed to see several students whom I recognized to have genetic diseases or other birth defect syndromes who had not been previously diagnosed.

It became clear to me that the staff of this wonderful facility was in need of some vital information about causes and treatments of children with mental handicaps. At that moment I decided to write this book, to serve as a guide to parents, educators, and other health care professionals who work with mentally handicapped children.

In order to provide optimal medical care and the best possible services to handicapped children, accurate medical diagnosis is crucial. The purpose of this book is to acquaint you with the many known causes, genetic and nongenetic, of mental dysfunction in children. This book will help you identify medical conditions that cause or contribute to mental disability and enable you to recognize children who could benefit from a genetic or medical evaluation. My emphasis on the importance of diagnosing these medical conditions may improve your understanding of children who have a diagnosis of a genetic disease or other medical problem and perhaps suggest new approaches to their education and treatment.

This book provides information for parents about what to do if you suspect that your child may have a mental or physical handicap to assure that the proper evaluations are performed and an appropriate treatment plan is developed.

Parents alone cannot provide all the diagnostic and therapeutic services necessary to provide optimum care for handicapped children. As parents, however, you need a way of assessing if your child is receiving the appropriate services from the appropriate professionals. This book will help you make these judgments and serve as a guide for your long journey with your child into adulthood.

Charles M. Strom

Chicago

Contents

Introduction

Two to three out of every hundred children will have difficulty progressing in the American educational system. These children may be classified as physically handicapped, mentally handicapped, or emotionally handicapped (Nelson, 1979, p. 158). Federal law has mandated that optimal educational and therapeutic services must be provided to these children (Wright, 1982; Cohen, 1982). Working with these children is simultaneously a rewarding and frustrating experience. Parents, teachers, therapists, school nurses, and school administrators must work together to provide the necessary services for handicapped children to optimize their development and education.

For about half of all severely mentally retarded children (I.Q. 40), it will be possible to identify a medical cause of their mental dysfunction (Kareggia et al., 1975; Gustavsonet et al., 1977; Laxova et al., 1977a,b). For children with more subtle forms of mental handicap, such as attention deficit disorder or learning disability, the percentage of children for whom a medical diagnosis can be established is much lower (Moser, Ramey, Leonard, 1983; Jones, 1988, pp. 618–622). The purpose of this book is to acquaint you with the many medical (genetic and nongenetic) causes of mental dysfunction in children and to alert you to certain signs and symptoms that may be indicative of a particular genetic problem.

Some of the causes of mental disability are preventable and some diseases are treatable. Throughout the book I stress the importance of early identification and diagnosis of these diseases.

In a recent study, 1 million consecutive births in British Columbia were surveyed. A total of 7.9% (approximately 79,000) of individuals under the age of 25 years had genetic diseases or other recognizable birth defects syndromes (Baird et al., 1988). Not all of these individuals had mental dysfunction as a result of their disorders; but these statistics reveal that genetic diseases and birth defect syndromes have a major impact on the health of a significant proportion of the population.

Perhaps as you read this book, some of you will recognize that your child or one of your students has symptoms of one of the diseases I describe; perhaps this will lead to a diagnosis and appropriate treatment for that child.

Why Is Establishing the Diagnosis of a Child Important?

Establishing an accurate medical diagnosis for a handicapped child is vitally important for the following reasons:

1. Knowing the correct diagnosis may, in some cases, lead to a specific treatment to alleviate some of the child's mental handicaps.
2. Knowing the correct diagnosis may lead to a more accurate prognosis for the future of a child.
3. Knowing the correct diagnosis may lead to medical intervention to prevent subsequent medical complications for the child.
4. Knowing the correct diagnosis may lead to the prediction of future progressive disability so that appropriate training can be introduced at an early age.
5. Knowing the correct diagnosis allows the prediction of the chances of parents having another child affected with the same problem, and allows calculation of the risks for other family members having a similarly affected child.
6. Knowing the correct diagnosis for a child may have important implications for the risks of that child eventually having children who are similarly affected.
7. Knowing the correct diagnosis is extremely helpful to parents and teachers who may be wondering why a child is having problems and helps to resolve the ambiguity and resultant anguish parents experience when they do not know "What is wrong with my child?"
8. Knowing the correct diagnosis can reassure parents about their adequacy as parents because it may reveal that their child's problems have a physical component and are not purely emotionally caused.

9. Knowing the correct diagnosis may lead to improved therapeutic interventions for the individual.
10. Knowing the correct diagnosis may be helpful in securing financial reimbursement for necessary services for an individual child.
11. Knowing the correct diagnosis can often lead to better awareness of the nature of a child's handicap, and can facilitate future treatment.
12. Knowing the correct diagnosis may allow participation in research protocols to evaluate new and experimental treatments.

Why Are Diagnoses Missed?

During my visit to the Laremont School, I was incredulous. I asked myself, "How can it be that the proper diagnoses for these children were missed?" On further reflection I could identify several reasons for this phenomenon.

Many of the adolescents in the Laremont School were last evaluated from the medical standpoint more than a decade ago. The progress of genetics has been so swift that more than 270 *new* genetic diseases have been identified since 1983. For example, Fragile X syndrome, the second most common genetic cause of mental retardation, (Down syndrome is the most common) hadn't been discovered 10 years ago. So, an adolescent boy who has not been evaluated in the last 10 years could not possibly have been appropriately tested and diagnosed for Fragile X syndrome.

Many genetic diseases impart unusual facial or physical characteristics to their sufferers. Often, however, these features are extremely subtle in infancy and become more pronounced as the child grows. Thus, though the diagnosis was missed in infancy, in adolescence the feature may be easily recognizable to a trained eye. This is why it is vital to reevaluate handicapped children annually.

There are well over 3000 different genetic diseases and birth defect syndromes. It is not reasonable to expect a general physician to be familiar with all of these disorders; most physicians who attended medical school before 1980 were probably not taught much about human genetics. The clinical specialities of genetics and dysmorphology, the study of birth defects, are relatively recent additions to the medical community. Referral patterns from general pediatricians, family practitioners, and general practitioners to geneticists and dysmorphologists are not well established. Many children with mental handicaps are either referred only to pediatric neurologists or are not referred to specialists at all. Therefore, many handicapped children have not received complete genetic evaluations.

For parents, caring for a handicapped child becomes a life-long crusade. After years of fruitless trips to doctors and specialists in search of the cause and cure for their child's handicap, parents may give up on the medical system. Parents may also be confused by educational and medical terminology. For example, parents may incorrectly believe that descriptive terms such as attention deficit disorder and learning disability constitute a medical diagnosis, when these terms describe specific educational problems. In such cases parents may think they have reached "the end of the road" and decide that no further medical evaluation is necessary or possible. This prevents establishing an accurate diagnosis.

For these reasons, I am certain that some children with genetic diseases and birth defect syndromes will continue to "slip through the cracks" and enter the school system without an accurate medical diagnosis of their problem.

I hope this book will help you, parents and educators, in your quest to provide optimal treatment for handicapped children in your care.

Chapter 1

IQ and Achievement Testing
What Does It Mean?

The subject of this chapter is intelligence testing (IQ) and the interpretation of the IQ test results. Although most of us know intuitively what "intelligence" is, the definition of intelligence is broadly debated in the scientific community. In a recent study (Snyderman and Rothman, 1987) 1020 experts in the fields of psychology, education, sociology, and genetics were asked what they considered to be the important aspects of intelligence. Almost all of the experts selected abstract reasoning, the capacity to acquire knowledge, and problem-solving ability as crucial components of intelligence. More than half of the experts also included adaptation to one's environment (social and interpersonal skills), creativity, general knowledge, linguistic competence, mathematical competence, memory, and mental speed as important features of intelligence.

Mental handicaps are defined largely by the results of standardized testing. The results of this testing will de-

termine the classification of a child's dysfunction, and therapeutic decisions and interventions will be based on this
classification. It is vital to understand how these tests are
designed, administered, and interpreted in order to understand the results.

It is important to keep in mind that many variables
are involved in determining the intelligence of any child.
His or her social and emotional capacities, as well as his
or her performance on standardized tests, go into a comprehensive assessment of intelligence. The diagnosis of
mental retardation and the label "mentally retarded"
should only be assigned to a child following an evaluation
of all the above listed aspects of intelligence, not solely
by his or her standardized test scores. Evaluation of all
the variables of intelligence requires not only standardized
testing but personal interviews with parents and teachers
and direct observations of the child at home and in school.

Thus, when I define IQ scores of between 55–69 as
the "mildly mentally retarded" range, this does not mean
that all children who score within this range are mentally
retarded. An individual child may score 68 and have excellent adaptive and social skills that place him in the "borderline intellectual functioning" category, a classification
that suggests stronger mental capacity than "mildly mentally retarded."

It is also important to note that there are different
standardized tests to measure intelligence, and numerical
scores vary slightly depending on the test. In this book,
I refer to the WISC-R, Wechsler Intelligence Test-Revised,
as the basis for the discussion of IQ testing.

Standardized testing is routinely used in the educational evaluation of children with possible mental handicaps. So, it is important to understand the terminology

used in reporting test results to interpret a child's test scores correctly. The terms normal, standard deviation, grade equivalence, age equivalence, and percentile rankings are discussed in this chapter. *Assessment of Children*, by Jerome Sattler (1988), is an excellent text to use to supplement the information given in this chapter.

Normal and Abnormal

The terms normal and abnormal have both common definitions and specific statistical definitions. I will put the word normal in quotation marks when using it in the common sense, that is, to refer to someone considered within the mainstream of the population. Italics are used to indicate the strict statistical meaning of a word.

Normal is defined statistically by measuring particular parameters, such as height, weight, or Intelligence Quotient (IQ), in large numbers of individuals. Since it is impossible to measure all members of a large society, scientists analyze a sample of the population.

In order to collect meaningful and valid data, a representative sample of all children, not just the "normal" ones, must be measured. The sample should include average children and gifted children, as well as mentally handicapped children. This is as it should be.

Once we are satisfied that the population we have chosen to study is truly representative of the population at large, we can call our population a *normal* population. A population that is not representative of the entire population is called a *skewed* population.

The most commonly used test for assessing intellectual function in children is the Intelligence Quotient (IQ).

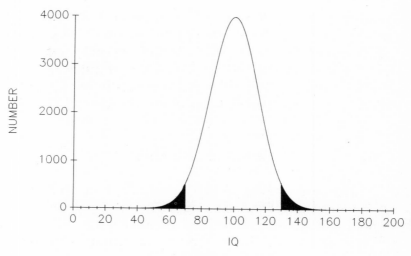

Figure 1

IQ tests are standardized tests administered to hundreds of thousands of children in the United States and in the industrialized world (Ramey & Finklestein, 1981; Moser, Ramey, & Leonard, 1983).

Once all the data have been collected, a *normal curve* is generated. This is a statistical term that refers to the graphical representation of all the scores in a given population. An idealized normal curve of IQ for a population is shown in Fig. 1. The vertical axis (up and down) represents the number of children with a given IQ, and the horizontal axis (side to side) represents the IQ. The curve is shaped like a bell; hence the term bell-shaped curve. The curve has this shape because 2.5% of children have IQs over 130, and 2.5% of children have IQs less than 70. Most children have IQs in the middle of this range (near 100). The average IQ (the sum of all the IQ scores divided by the number of children tested) is called the *mean* in statistical terms. For IQ testing the mean is defined as a score of 100. The mean is the same as the "average." Another statistical term that describes the center of this curve is the term *median*. The median is defined as the IQ score that half of all children scored below and half of all children scored above. Usually the median and the mean are very close. Another way to describe the median is the term 50th percentile. The 50th percentile is identical to the median, it is the score that 50% of children score above and 50% of children score below. The mean (average) and median (50th percentile) are measurements that indicate the center (middle) of the normal curve. For IQ testing, the mean is defined as a score of 100 whereas the median will be somewhere close to 100.

Another vital fact to know about IQ scores is how much these scores vary among all the children tested. Several other statistical terms are required to describe fully our normal curve. The *range* of test scores is simply the highest to the lowest score for all the tests. On our graph, the IQ scores range from a low of 35 to a high of 145. Therefore the *range* is 35–145. For the purposes of understanding your child's scores, statistical calculations made of the variability of test scores for all the children (not just the highest and lowest) are the most important. These numbers are a reflection of how widely individuals vary within a population. Although these numbers go by various names—standard deviation or standard error of the mean—they are all measuring the same thing, namely, how widely did the children vary in their test scores. On a normal curve, the distance of any score from the mean can be measured in several ways.

IQ scores are reported in a special way. An IQ of

Table 1. Scores in Relation to Mental Function*

Less than 25	Profound mental retardation
25–39	Severe mental retardation
40–54	Moderate mental retardation
55–69	Mild mental retardation
70–80	Borderline intellectual functioning
80–90	Low average intelligence
90–115	Average intelligence
115–130	High average intelligence
More than 130	Gifted–superior

*Based on WISC-R (Sattler, 1988).

100 is defined as the mean and each 15 points above or below 100 represents approximately one standard deviation. Therefore a score of 115 is 1 standard deviation above the median and 85 is 1 standard deviation below the median. By definition 95% of all children will fall within the limits of 2 standard deviations below the mean (IQ = 70) and 2 standard deviation above the mean (IQ = 130). Each range of IQ has a description. These are listed in Table 1.

Children with IQs between 70 and 80 are not considered to be mentally retarded. However, children with borderline intellectual functioning will be noticeably slower than other children with respect to grasping new ideas and achieving well in school. Such children need tutoring to progress in school with their peers.

Mildly retarded children (IQs 55–69) can usually learn to read, write and perform simple calculations if no other physical or emotional problems are present. The adult educational achievement level for mildly retarded children is usually a 3rd–5th grade level. These children are described as being *educable* because of their ability to learn rudimentary academic skills.

Mildly retarded children who have no other physical or emotional problems will be able to learn to dress themselves, wash themselves, be toilet-trained and, in general, function independently in daily skills. This is described as *trainable*. The ultimate goal for a mildly retarded child is to live independently from his or her parents in a sheltered environment and to work in unskilled and semi-skilled positions. This goal is not easily attained and its accomplishment requires tremendous effort from the child, his parents, and professionals. Thus mildly retarded children are considered to be *trainable and educable*. Mental age at adulthood will range from 8 years to 11 years old.

Moderately retarded children are considered *trainable but not educable*. With tremendous effort, children with IQ scores between 40–54 may eventually learn to read and write at a first-grade level. Their vocational potential is limited to sheltered workshop environments and these children will require supervised living environments throughout their lives. The average mental age at adulthood will be between 6 and 8 years old.

Severely and profoundly retarded children will usually be unable to acquire any academic skills and usually require institutionalization or closely supervised home care.

Approximately 3% (3 per hundred) of all children will be mentally retarded. In the United States, where there are approximately 3 million births per year, about 90,000 mentally retarded children are born every year. A breakdown of numbers in each category of mental retardation appears in Table 2.

IQ testing can usually be performed reliably at any time after the age of 2 years. The most commonly ad-

Table 2. Mental Retardation

Total	3%	90,000/year*
Mild	2.7	81,000/year
Moderate	0.2	6,000/year
Severe/profound	0.15	4,500/year

*Adapted from Sattler, 1988, p. 648.

ministered IQ tests are the Stanford-Binet and the Wechsler tests. There are several Wechsler tests which are administered to children at different ages. The Wechsler tests are composed of a combination of several subtests. Each test attempts to measure a particular aspect of intelligence, for example vocabulary, spelling, or letter writing. A child is given a score for each of the subtests in addition to three cumulative scores. The three cumulative scores are called the *Verbal IQ*, which measures verbal intelligence, *Performance IQ*, which measures nonverbal intelligence, and *Full Scale IQ*, which combines both the Verbal and the Performance IQ into a final score (Sattler, 1988).

All the scores (all subtests, Verbal IQ, Performance IQ, and Full Scale IQ) for mentally retarded children will be similar. IQ testing is specifically designed to be independent of age or educational achievement. Theoretically, your child's IQ should be exactly the same at 10 years of age as it is at 16 years of age. If your child experiences more than a 10-point loss of IQ points, a medical evaluation should be performed immediately to make sure that the child is not suffering from a medical condition causing mental deterioration.

Normal is defined medically as an individual whose measured value fits within an arbitrary range. For example, for IQ, all children whose intelligence is between 2 standard deviations below the mean and 2 standard deviations above the mean (shaded area on Fig. 1) are considered of normal intelligence. In contrast, any child whose IQ is less than 2 standard deviations below the mean or more than 2 standard deviations above the mean is considered *abnormal.*

Therefore, the determination of whether or not a given measurement for any child is normal or abnormal depends on his status with respect to the normal curve established for that particular measurement (in this example, IQ).

All other forms of academic testing involve the assessment of the achievement of various skills. This kind of testing is called *achievement testing;* it examines cumulative academic accomplishments such as math and reading skills. Unlike IQ testing, achievement test results vary with age and education. A child will score better on a reading comprehension test in the third grade than on a similar test taken in the first grade.

Most achievement tests are standardized. A *standardized* achievement test takes into account age variability in test scores. The results of a standardized test for a first-grader will indicate how a child's skills compare with respect to all other first graders in the country (or state, or school). Standardized achievement test scores are often reported in terms of *percentiles.* A child who scores in the 90th percentile for his age has scored higher than 90% of his classmates and lower than 10% of his classmates. A student scoring in the 10th percentile has scored lower than 90% of his classmates and higher than 10% of his classmates.

Another way of reporting standardized test scores is

in terms of *grade equivalent* or age equivalent. Grade equivalent means that a child's score is equal to the average score for all children in that grade. A fourth grader who reads at a sixth-grade equivalent is doing well. If he reads at a first-grade level he is delayed, and if he reads at a fourth-grade level he is "grade appropriate." *Age equivalent* is an analogous term used for preschool children or for reporting nonacademic skills.

The three most common ways to express the results of achievement tests are raw scores, percentiles, and grade or age equivalents. Age equivalents are used for preschool children and grade equivalents are used for school-aged children. When attempting to understand your child's test scores, it is a good idea to ignore the "raw" scores. Raw test scores vary from test to test seemingly without rhyme or reason, and are difficult for a nonexpert to understand. The helpful scores are the standardized scores, which are reported in percentiles, grade or age equivalences, or both.

When examining percentile scores, it is important to determine the population of students with whom your child's score is being compared. For example, a particular child in an affluent suburban school district may score in the 30th percentile (that is, he has scored higher than 30% of children in the United States and lower than 70%) when compared to the entire United States but only in the 10th percentile (lower than 90%) for his school or school district. Often I am asked to evaluate a child for learning disabilities or mental retardation who is of average intelligence but is in an extremely high-powered academic placement.

Grade or age equivalence is the grade or age when your child's score is the 50th percentile. If your child is in the 6th grade and scores at a 6th-grade equivalent, he

Table 3. Test Scores of Three 6th-Grade Children

	Average	Gifted	Retarded
Raw score: (ignore)	500	780	250
Percentile	50th	99th	3rd
Grade equivalent	6th	9th	3rd

is performing as expected. Again, it is important to find out what population your child is being compared to in order to make an accurate assessment. As an example, let us look at the test scores of three 6th-grade children; an "average" child, a gifted child, and a mildly retarded child. The scores for these children expressed in various ways are tabulated in Table 3.

The average child is scoring higher than half his classmates and lower than half his classmates. His scores put him in the 50th percentile of 6th graders, so his grade equivalence is 6th grade.

The gifted child has scored higher than 99% of his classmates and his scores would put him in the 50th percentile in the 9th grade.

The mildly retarded child, however, has scored lower than 97% of his classmates and is functioning at an equivalent to an average third-grader.

Mental retardation and learning disability are for the most part defined by IQ testing. Mentally retarded children usually have a Verbal IQ, Performance IQ, and Full-Scale IQ below 70. Learning-disabled children will have a Full-Scale IQ of more than 80, and the subtest scores should define a specific area or areas of disability (see Chapter 2). We can now discuss other terms used to describe mentally handicapped children.

Chapter 2

Mental Dysfunction
Definition of Terms

Infant Development

The term *infant development* is used to describe the predictable, progressive attainment of skills by children. The skills of rolling over, sitting, crawling, walking, talking, drinking from a cup, climbing stairs, and riding a bicycle are all examples of infant developmental skills. These skills are also called developmental milestones.

Abnormal patterns of development in infants and children with mental dysfunction often provide clues to the etiology of their handicap. The terms *failure to thrive, developmental delay, mental retardation, learning disability, loss of developmental milestones, attention deficit disorder, hypotonia of infancy, emotional disability, conduct disability, autism, and mental illness* are specific terms with specific definitions and should not be used interchangeably. An older term, minimal brain dysfunction, is no longer useful.

This chapter contains definitions for these terms and concludes with a classification scheme I use in a medical evaluation of a child with mental handicap. It does not replace psychologists' and educators' more elaborate classification schemes formulated for the purposes of designing educational strategies for handicapped children. Sattler's textbook is an excellent resource for those wishing more information regarding developmental testing and evaluation.

Physical versus Intellectual Function

An evaluation of an infant or toddler for a potential mental or physical handicap begins with an examination of his or her performance of certain age-appropriate skills, such as sitting up, walking, or speaking in sentences. These skills, attained by all "normal" children in a predictable sequence, are called *developmental milestones.*

Motor milestones involve the combined action of the brain, nerves, and muscles. Rolling over, grasping objects, transferring objects from one hand to the other, walking, running, athletic ability, coordination, and strength are examples of primarily physical or motor skills. The term *developmental delay* is used to describe children who are delayed in developing motor milestones.

Intellectual milestones primarily involve the high-level functioning of the brain. Reading, writing, mathematics, social skills, thinking, and planning are all examples of primarily intellectual skills. The objective measurement of intellectual functioning is the Intelligence Quotient, or IQ (see Chapter 1).

Studies observing several thousand children (including gifted and handicapped children) have established normal standards for the age when children attain developmental milestones. As in all such measurements there is variability among different children. For example, one child may begin walking at 10 months of age and another at 14 months of age. Statistical analyses predict a *normal range* of ages for attainment of each milestone. These calculations are called *normal standards*. As we discussed, normal is a statistical term that means that statistical calculations have been made for an entire population to obtain ranges and statistical variability.

If a child has not attained a developmental milestone by the age when 95% of children attain that milestone, then, by statistical definition, the child is *delayed* for that milestone. If several milestones are delayed in a child, the term *developmental delay* is appropriate.

Normal standard calculations allow us to say that 95% of all children will be walking by the age 18 months. If a child is not walking by that time, this milestones is described as being delayed in this child. It is important to note that age cut-offs for the attainment of milestone are calculated statistically. Because of this there will *always* be 5% of the population of children defined as delayed for each milestone; when statistical calculations are performed, the first 95% of children who attain a milestone are *defined* as being normal. Therefore 5% of children will always be defined as being delayed for each milestone.

If all children began walking at earlier ages, the calculations would simply reduce the age limit from 18 months to an earlier time and 5% of children would still be considered delayed.

Fortunately, the standard values for child development have not varied appreciably in the past two decades. However, for some measurements such as height the normal curves are continually changing. Children in the United States are consistently taller than the previous generation.

A rough estimate of a child's achievement of developmental milestones can be accomplished by a pediatrician when he or she asks parents questions and performs a routine examination of the child. If there is a question of a possible developmental delay, a more extensive examination by a specialist in childhood development should be performed. This examination is called a *developmental examination* and can be performed by a pediatric neurologist, a pediatric developmental specialist, clinical psychologist, occupational therapist, or physical therapist. In my experience, the quality of the developmental examination is less affected by the degree of the examiner than by his or her acumen, interest, and experience. The examiner will choose the appropriate test or tests for each individual child. Two of the most popular tests are called the *Denver Developmental Test* and the *Bayley Developmental Tests*.

The results of the standardized tests are usually reported in age-equivalences: for example, a 14-month-old child may be functioning at a 9-month-old level.

If the developmental examination confirms the suspicions regarding delayed attainment of milestones, the child should undergo a special examination by a pediatric neurologist. This examination, called a *neurological examination*, is to determine if there are any physical signs and symptoms of brain dysfunction. The neurological examination may reveal an abnormality such as spasticity (increased muscle tone), hypotonia (poor muscle tone), or poor coordination.

At this point a genetic evaluation is also warranted to determine if there is a genetic disease or multiple malformation syndrome present.

To attain appropriate developmental milestones and to have a normal neurological examination, a child must have normal functioning of his brain, nerves, and muscles.

Because an infant cannot talk or follow directions, his or her developmental progress is monitored almost entirely by the motor milestones. It is impossible to administer an IQ test to a newborn. Nonverbal tests designed to estimate intellectual functioning are available to assess children in infancy and toddlerhood. These tests are extremely difficult to administer and interpret and they require normal functioning of muscles and nerves in a child to give accurate results. Standardized IQ testing becomes reliable after two years of age (see Chapter 1). It is also impossible to administer the standard Denver Developmental Test of infant development to a baby who is paralyzed, since this test primarily examines physical skills. These represent the two extremes in differences between physical (or motor) development and intellectual development. It is often difficult to separate purely intellectual functioning from motor functioning in infants and toddlers.

The first evidence of *intellectual* dysfunction is often the observation of developmental delay. However, it is important to understand that *not all children with developmental delay will grow up to be mentally retarded, and vice versa*. For example, children with congenital muscular dystrophy, a muscle disease causing progressive muscle weakness during infancy, often show severe developmental delay in motor skill attainment. Affected children may never stand or walk, but these children usually have completely normal intellectual functioning throughout life. They have severe developmental delay without mental retardation.

It is also possible for a child with mild mental retardation to attain motor skills within the normal time sequence. The significance of a child's inability to perform a particular skill will depend on the total medical and physical condition of the child. Some children with severe learning problems may appear completely "normal" until they begin school.

The prognosis for a child with developmental delay is quite variable. Some children with a disorder known as benign hypotonia of infancy will "outgrow" their problems and live lives without mental handicap. For other children, developmental delay will be the first sign of a serious or even lethal disease, with profound implications for their futures.

In order to establish a prognosis for a child with developmental delays, the appropriate evaluations need to be performed. Developmental testing, neurological examination and evaluation, and genetic examination and evaluation should be performed. The genetic and/or neurological evaluations may discover the cause for the delay, in which case a prognosis will be possible.

If no diagnosis can be made immediately, children with delayed development should be followed at six-month intervals by the specialists so that their patterns of handicap can be determined and appropriate therapies can be prescribed.

Developmental delays in children are variable in patterns, and in time. Analysis of the patterns of delays often shed important light on a child's problems. For example, a child who is not walking at 14 months of age but is speaking 50 words and responding to commands is less at risk for future intellectual handicaps than a child of the same age who is neither walking nor talking.

In addition, the magnitude of the delays are important. A child who is only a few months late to develop milestones has a better prognosis than a child consistently a year late for the same milestones.

Few skills can be described as either purely intellectual or purely physical. Reading is a good example of a skill that is almost totally intellectual. The only physical requirement to read is good vision.

Speech is an example of another primarily intellectual skill but also requires normal functioning of the mouth, tongue, vocal cords, and cerebellum (the part of the brain responsible for coordination). The child's brain must learn how to interpret and initiate speech, but the muscles of the tongue, mouth, and vocal cords must perform the skill. Any hearing impairment will also lead to deficiencies in speech development.

Delayed speech is very often the first indication that a child has an intellectual handicap. As soon as the delay is noticed, complete evaluations by a speech therapist and physician are necessary to determine if there are any physical reasons for the lack of speech. These evaluations will include hearing tests and examination of the muscles involved in the production of speech. If no physical handicaps are discovered, the delayed speech is probably the first sign of an intellectual handicap (either mental retardation or learning disability).

Examples of how mistakes can be made in interpreting developmental problems are illustrated in the following cases.

Children with a *biochemical disease* called multiple carboxylase deficiency (see p. 187) can have severe developmental delay. If the diagnosis is not made these children may not roll over, sit up or walk. However, if the diagnosis is made, these children can be treated with a vitamin called biotin. After treatment these children begin to develop normally and have normal intellectual functioning. Children with this disease can be inappropriately labeled mentally retarded when in fact they have normal intelligence. The appropriate term for these children is developmentally delayed, not mentally retarded.

As mentioned previously, children with certain forms of muscular dystrophy can have extreme developmental delays due to weakness of their muscles. Children with some forms of muscular dystrophy may never be able to sit up without assistance, but have completely normal intellectual functioning. Again the term developmental delay is the appropriate term for these children. Children with congenital muscular dystrophy can be recognized by abnormalities in their neurological examination.

Children with *dyslexia*, an isolated problem involving an inability to learn to read and write, often have completely normal development. Thus normal development is no guarantee that a child will have no mental dysfunction, just as developmental delay is no guarantee that a child will have subsequent mental dysfunction.

Hypotonia in Infancy

Hypotonia is a medical term used to refer to infants who have poor muscle tone. Hypotonia is diagnosed by neurological examination. Analogous to developmental delay, poor muscle tone can be caused by many different problems, only one of which is mental retardation. Hypotonia can be caused by diseases affecting the muscles, such as muscular dystrophy, diseases affecting the brain, severe brain damage, or biochemical abnormalities that interfere with normal functioning of the nerves or the brain.

The evaluation of a child with hypotonia in infancy is extremely complex and beyond the scope of this discussion. The ultimate prognosis for a child with hypotonia in infancy can vary from completely normal (benign hypotonia of infancy) to death in infancy. Even after extensive evaluations, it may be impossible to determine the exact prognosis for a given child before the child is observed over a period of several months, or even years. A child with hypotonia needs close neurological follow-up.

A history of hypotonia in infancy is always significant in a child who subsequently develops a mental handicap. These children are almost certain to have a medical cause for their mental dysfunction.

Loss of Developmental Milestones

This term refers to children who have successfully attained a developmental milestone and then lose their ability to perform the same task. True *loss of developmental milestones* must be distinguished from temporary regres-

sion. In the presence of stress (either emotional or physical) children may "regress" to a prior developmental
stage. For example, a young child experiencing stress (i.e.,
divorce, moving to another city, or death of a loved one)
can, temporarily, lose the developmental milestone of toilet training and begin having urinary or stool "accidents."

A child who regresses will regain the lost skills within
a short period of time with the appropriate psychological
support. Children with true loss of milestones never regain
a skill once they have lost it. The loss of milestones and
mental deterioration may be very gradual, but is progressive, so that as the child gets older he loses more and
more of his abilities. It is possible to be fooled into thinking that a child is regressing, when, in fact, he or she is
losing milestones.

Learning Disabilities (Excluding Attention Deficit Disorder)

In the most general sense, a *learning disability* (LD)
can be defined as any dysfunction that interferes with the
normal accumulation of intellectual skills. By definition, a
learning disabled child is one for whom testing reveals a
normal Intelligence Quotient (IQ) and who is unable to
function well in a mainstream classroom (Cruikshank,
1977).

The definition of learning disability is determined by
the results of educational testing. In order to understand
the concept of a learning disability it is important to discuss the interpretation of the most popular tests in use
today. For children under the age of 16, the most commonly administered test is called the Wechsler Intelligence

Scale-Revised or the WISC-R. This test is divided into 12 segments called subtests. Each subtest is designed to measure a particular aspect of intelligence.

The subtests of the WISC-R are Information, Similarities, Arithmetic, Vocabulary, Comprehension, Digit Span, Picture Completion, Picture Arrangement, Block Design, Object Assembly, Coding, and Mazes. The first six subtests listed measure verbal skills, and the last six measure nonverbal skills. For Information, Similarities, Arithmetic, Vocabulary, and Comprehension, the examiner reads questions to the child and writes down the oral responses. In the Digit Span subtest, the child is asked to repeat a series of numbers read by the examiner. In the Picture Completion subtest the child is shown drawings with critical features missing and is asked to tell the examiner what is needed to properly complete the drawing. In the Picture Arrangement subtest, the child is asked to arrange a series of pictures into a logical progression. In the Block Design subtest the child is asked to arrange colored blocks to match a pattern. In the Object Assembly subtest the child is given pieces of an object and asked to arrange them into a meaningful object (similar to a simple jigsaw puzzle). In the Coding subtest the child is given a simple object code (for example a diamond shape equalling 2) and is asked to copy the appropriate symbol under the number. In the Mazes subtest, the child is asked to complete a series of mazes. Each subtest has a time limit for completion.

The final testing report may be lengthy and may be difficult for a layperson to understand. However, there are three numbers to look for that measure a student's Intelligence Quotient (IQ). These are the verbal IQ, the performance IQ, and the full scale IQ. The *verbal* IQ is an average of all the verbal subtests, the *performance* IQ is an average of the nonverbal subtests, and the *full scale* IQ score is a combination of the verbal and performance scores.

For all IQ scores, 100 is the average for the entire population (see Chapter 1).

IQ testing, as noted, is independent of age. A child should have the same IQ at 6 as he has at 16 (see Chapter 1).

A child with a learning disability has an IQ score above the borderline range (more than 69), but has deficiencies defined by his performance on the various subtests. The analysis of the subtest results often points to specific areas of weakness (disability), and provides the basis for designing an appropriate treatment plan for a given child.

Let's look at some examples of test scores of four children.

Frank was first tested at 10 years of age. He was referred for learning disability evaluation because he was doing poorly in school. His teacher complained that he was inattentive to tasks, fidgeted in his seat, and continually disrupted her classroom.

Frank's testing revealed that his verbal IQ was 87 whereas his performance IQ was 105, yielding a full-scale IQ of 96. Frank is of normal intelligence, but the analysis of his subtest scores revealed the reasons for his difficulty in school. Although he was reading at grade level (in the fourth grade), his ability to process and understand language was impaired. He was able to compensate reasonably well because his abilities to reason and understand concepts were intact. Frank's inattentive behavior in class was a defensive diversion, unconsciously developed to hide his disability. His teacher thought he wasn't trying, but in reality, Frank *couldn't* produce the expected schoolwork. Children with undiagnosed learning disabilities are often described by the teacher as highly distractible, lazy, and immature. A child who seems bright but "can't concentrate" or is described in the above terms should be referred for learning disability testing immediately. Unlike mentally retarded children, learning-disabled children often suffer problems of low self-esteem because they are acutely aware of disappointing teachers and parents.

With tutoring and the aid of a word processor, Frank has done better in school. Sessions with a child psychiatrist were crucial because Frank had developed a poor self image. Therapy sessions really helped Frank to understand his disability and to feel better about himself. Within a few months of his diagnosis, the behavior problems diminished considerably and his academic performance has improved markedly. This is an example of how prompt intervention, good testing, and appropriate therapy completely turned around a boy's life.

Alexandra is a 14-year-old girl whom I evaluated for a possible learning disability. She attended a high-powered academic private school and she was getting Cs and Ds in her classes. Her testing revealed a performance IQ of 88, a verbal IQ of 91 and a full-scale IQ of 90. The subtest scores revealed that she had no outstanding strengths or weaknesses. All of Alexandra's scores were around 90. (This is in contrast to Frank, whose performance scores were 18 points lower than his verbal scores and where the subtests revealed specific weaknesses).

I informed Alexandra's parents that she did not have

a learning disability. She was of average intelligence without any particular disabilities. Alexandra's "problem" was that she was placed in classes for extremely bright children in a very competitive academic setting. In a school with a curriculum designed for average students, Alexandra would perform better. I tried, in vain, to convince her parents to transfer Alexandra to a public school or to a private school program that was less demanding.

Tony, an 8-year-old boy, was also tested for learning disabilities. The testing revealed an almost total inability to read or to write sentences. This led to a diagnosis of dyslexia. Dyslexia is one of the most common forms of learning disability. It is a mysterious disorder in which individuals have extreme difficulty reading and writing. Dyslexia is five times more common in boys than girls. Sometimes the dyslexia is so severe that affected children simply *can't* ever be taught to read. Usually, with intensive remediation, dyslexic children can be taught to read at a basic level.

If Tony's dyslexia had remained undiagnosed, a tragic spiral could begin. In school, teachers would keep trying to teach him how to read and he would continue to fail. His self-image would be poor because he would see himself failing every day. School would become hateful and he might eventually drop out.

For Tony, the appropriate diagnosis and treatment of his dyslexia interrupted this spiral. He can have books read to him, and he can answer test questions orally. Books are available on tape for dyslexic individuals and for the blind.

One of my classmates at Yale who could barely write his name because of dyslexia was able to graduate in 4 years using his tape recorder extensively to "take notes," listen to reading material, and take examinations. He also received help from friends who read material to him.

Esther is a 6-year-old girl-referred to me by her kindergarten teacher because of concerns regarding her ability to succeed in first grade. Although she tried very hard in class, she was not developing the cognitive skills expected of kindergartners.

Esther's IQ scores are all around 68. She does not have a learning disability but is classified as mildly mentally retarded (see Table 1). However, testing was useful in designing tutoring programs to take advantage of her relative strengths and to help improve her weaknesses.

Attention Deficit Disorder

Attention deficit disorder can be a catchall description. With a school-aged child the term is usually used to describe a child with a very short attention span in school and who is easily distractible. Children may or may not have a "hyperactive" component to their attention deficit disorder. This is manifested by an inability to sit for reasonable periods at a desk, and/or by disruptive physical behavior. Usually pre-school children are identified as having attention deficit disorder because of "hyperactive" behavior. Children with attention deficit disorders are often classified as learning disabled, and vice versa. For example, Frank could easily have been labeled with attention deficit disorder if his learning disability had gone undetected.

There are many different causes (medical, genetic, and emotional) for attention deficit disorders. If your child is labeled with attention deficit disorder, a complete learning disability and medical evaluation is advisable immediately.

Minimal Brain Dysfunction

Prior to the development of the concepts of learning disabilities and attention deficit disorder, professionals were intrigued by children with such subtle forms of mental handicaps. Many articles were written about children affected with these problems who often had so-called "soft" neurological signs. These soft neurological signs were subtle abnormalities in the neurological examinations. It was then extrapolated that these children, whom we now classify as learning-disabled with or without attention deficit disorders, must have some subtle form of brain damage. The term *minimal brain dysfunction* was coined to describe such children with subtle mental handicaps and soft neurological signs.

The term minimal brain dysfunction is no longer useful for several reasons. The diagnosis of minimal brain dysfunction leads to no specific intervention or prognosis. There is no concrete evidence that children classified as having minimal brain dysfunction actually have any physical brain damage, and there are now specific diagnoses and etiologies defined for such children.

Emotional Disability

This term refers to a child who has problems interacting with others. Symptoms of children with *emotional diabilities* vary widely among different children. Some children will be excessively shy and withdrawn. Others will act inappropriately towards others. Some will be depressed or develop eating disorders resulting in obesity or anorexia nervosa (extreme loss of weight).

Emotional disorders can be caused by other medical or mental problems. For example, learning disabilities often cause emotional problems in children. A child who is diagnosed as having an emotional disability should *always* have a complete learning disability evaluation, medical evaluation, and genetic evaluation, in addition to a psychological evaluation to investigate the possibility that the emotional disability may be caused by a learning disability or medical problem. It is common to blame family stresses for emotional disturbances, but all children (and parents) deserve the benefit of the doubt. If the emotional disability is the result of another problem, both problems must be treated.

Conduct Disturbance

Conduct disturbance is an extreme example of an emotional disability. Children with a conduct disturbance are continually disruptive in the classroom and act aggressively toward other children. These children usually require special classrooms that use behavior modification techniques (see below) to control the disruptive behavior. As in emotional disability, children with conduct disorders should have a complete learning disability, neurologic, and genetic evaluation to ascertain if another problem is contributing to the conduct problem.

Mental Illness

Mental illness is a general term I will use in this book to describe children and adolescents with incapacitating mental problems. Another word for mental illness used in this context is psychosis. There are three major classification of mental illness.

1. Thought disorders (schizophrenia)
2. Unipolar disorders (depression)
3. Bipolar disorders (manic-depression)

The onset of *schizophrenia* commonly occurs in adolescence. Young men or women may suddenly have a "mental breakdown" or "nervous breakdown" and require hospitalization. The medical term for this is psychotic break. Adolescents with schizophrenia will usually require specific antipsychotic medication. Thorazine, Mellaril, Haldol, and Stelazine are examples of such medication. Unipolar disorder or depression is not depression that is a normal part of the ups and downs of life. Unipolar depression is an incapacitating illness. People are unable to get out of bed or function in society. Treatment for depression usually involves medications called antidepressants. Tofranil, Elavil, and Sinequan are examples of antidepressant medications.

Bipolar disorder, or *manic-depressive disorder*, involves fluctuations from periods of being "high" with periods of depression. During periods of mood elevation (called hypomanic episodes) the individuals feel invincible and on top of the world. People in manic episodes often make impulsive business or personal decisions because of their feelings of invulnerability. After a period of time (usually several days to several weeks) people come down from the high and crash into a depression. The usual treatment for bipolar disorder is a drug called Lithium, although sometimes antidepressant agents are used instead.

These forms of mental illness are diseases that have both a genetic component and an environmental component. There are three genetic diseases that can cause mental illness, namely, Klinefelter's syndrome, XYY syndrome (Chapter 6), and Wilson's disease (Chapter 8). Every adolescent with mental illness should be evaluated for these diseases.

Autism

Five out of every 10,000 infants will suffer from a severe form of mental dysfunction known as *autism*. Autism afflicts boys 3–4 times more often than girls. There are four aspects to the diagnosis of autism. A review of these aspects is contained in an excellent two-article series by Minshew and Payton (1988a,b).

1. Marked inability to interact with other people (both other children and adults).
2. Delay in the development of normal speech.
3. Marked restriction in the range of interests.
4. Onset during infancy or childhood.

Autistic infants often stiffen while being held instead of cuddling their bodies into their parents'. They often prefer to be left alone. They develop attachments to inanimate objects, such as chairs or rulers rather than to parents, brothers, and sisters, blankets, stuffed animals, or dolls. They often perform rocking or head-banging in infancy (self-stimulatory behavior). (It is important to note that children who display some self-stimulatory behavior are not necessarily autistic.) Early in their speech development they only echo exactly what is said to them, with a monotone expression (echolalia).

The cause of autism is unknown, but there is increasing evidence that it is a physical problem and not caused by poor parenting. Until recently, autism was blamed on parents who were described as being extremely distant and cold with their children. The phrase "refrigerator parents" was coined to describe these parents whose lack of affection caused their children to be come autistic (Kanner, 1943, 1952).

We now know that this concept is false and has done a great disservice to parents of autistic children. It is difficult to care for a child who stiffens when being held and takes no comfort from hearing his parents' voices or seeing his parents' faces. The "refrigerator parents" behavior may have been the result of trying to raise an autistic child, not the cause of the autism.

The prognosis for autistic children varies with their intelligence. Some estimates are that 70% of autistic children are mentally retarded. The prognosis for retarded autistic children is poor. They may never develop normal speech or learn to interact with others.

Autistic children without retardation are also called "high-functioning autistics." These children eventually learn to hold conversations and can be taught the rudiments of social interactions. These children often develop a fixation with a particular narrow field of knowledge. For example, one boy memorized all the statistics from major-league baseball. He knew all the batting averages and standings for the past 50 years. When asked about the rules of the game, however, he knew nothing about baseball itself. These children are sometimes referred to as savants (formerly idiot-savants). The movie *Rain Man* portrayed an autistic savant with amazing mathematical powers.

Autistic children and adults are extremely dependent on routine. Unless everything is done exactly the same way every day, a tantrum or total disorientation results. One autistic child had a screaming tantrum for no apparent reason. Eventually it was determined that one book had been removed from a bookshelf containing more than 30 books in his room. He didn't read the books but he knew how many books were on the shelf and noticed that one was missing. This single disruption was sufficient to cause a major outburst from this patient.

Three diseases can cause autistic-like behavior and lead to the inappropriate diagnosis of autism. The X-linked genetic disease called the *Fragile X syndrome* (see Chapter 6) can cause autistic-like behavior. *Rett's syndrome* and *Cornelia de Lange syndrome* are also capable of causing behavior resembling autism. Unrecognized deafness in childhood can also cause autistic-like symptoms. With these exceptions, however, the cause of autism is not known. Clearly, bad parenting is *not* the cause, but the actual cause of autism is yet to be discovered.

There is no established specific medication for the treatment of autistic children. A new medication called fenfluramine has been shown to reduce hyperactivity and stereotyped behaviors in about one third of autistic children. Children with higher IQ's responded the best to

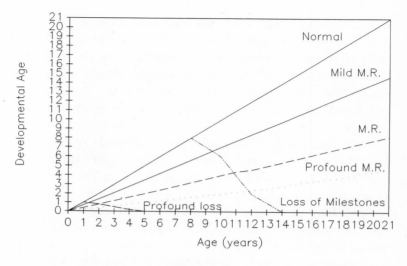

Figure 2

fenfluramine. Since this is a new drug, the possible side effects of long term use have not yet been established (for review, see du Verglas, Banks, and Guyer, 1988).

Behavior modification techniques (see Chapter 12) are currently the therapy of choice available for autistic children. It is possible for high-functioning autistics to live independently, but this is the exception rather than the rule.

A Model of Normal and Abnormal Development

Figure 2 is a graph of my model for the various forms of normal and abnormal development. The horizontal axis represents chronological time and the vertical axis represents developmental and intellectual functioning. On this graph, I assume that developmental delays observed in infancy indicate poor brain development leading to mental retardation. As discussed, this is usually, but not always, the case.

The line marked "normal" represents children who function at an age appropriate level at every age. In 1 year they attain the skills expected for that period of development. This graph does not show developmental spurts, times when developmental milestones are accrued at faster rates than at others. For example, in the period of time between 1 year and 2 years of age most children attain many developmental milestones. They begin to walk, talk, and feed themselves. In contrast, in the period between 2 and 3 years of age, children continue to progress, but their attainment of milestones is not as dramatic as in the previous year. First grade is another time when many milestones are attained.

The line labeled "Mild MR" represents a child with mild mental retardation. As you can see, in the first year of life the differences between the development of a mildly retarded child and a normal child are very small. Because there is a range of development among normal children, it is often impossible to predict whether a particular developmental lag is significant or whether it is simply an individual variation. For example, by the age of 14 months, 90% of all children will be walking. If walking is the only delay in a child, there may be no predictive significance to this lag. However, by 14 months a child should also be saying ma-ma or da-da specifically to indicate his or her parents, be able to drink from a cup, use a pincer grasp, and play pat-a-cake. There must be more concern for a child who is delayed in developing all of these skills than for a child with an isolated delay of one or two of them.

The gap between the skills attained by the normal child and the mildly retarded child broadens with time. Children who were not much different from other children in infancy and toddlerhood become increasingly delayed after school begins. Retarded children progress, but they do so at a slower rate, and with much more effort from their parents, teachers, and themselves.

In addition, when normal children enter periods of developmental spurts, the gap between mildly retarded children and their normal peers may seem to widen suddenly. First grade is such a time. A mildly retarded child may have been able to attend mainstream preschool and kindergarten but may be incapable of functioning in a mainstream first-grade classroom.

Following that year, he or she may no longer be able to socialize or play with the same friends as in the past. Although this may seem like a sudden deterioration, it is simply the natural result of the broadening gap between retarded children and their unaffected peers.

The line labeled "MR" represents a child with moderate mental retardation. This could describe a typical child with Down syndrome. Even in infancy, the developmental progress of children with moderate mental retardation is noticeably delayed. For example, a typical child with Down syndrome begins walking at 2–3 years of age. The gap between such children and their normal peers broadens much earlier and at a faster rate than for mildly retarded children. The eventual adult intellectual functioning for such a child is equivalent to that of an 8-year-old.

The line labeled "profound MR" shows a typical developmental profile of a profoundly retarded child. These children usually show abnormalities upon neurological examination and a near total lack of milestone attainment.

The curve labeled "profound loss" is an example of children who have diseases causing loss of developmental milestones. These disorders are discussed in detail in Chapter 7. Such children develop normally, or near-normally for a period of time, and then begin to lose skills they have already developed. This curve could represent the development of a child with the genetic disease Tay-Sachs disease. These children appear completely normal at birth and in early infancy. Usually, by a year of age, children with Tay-Sachs disease begin to deteriorate neurologically until death prior to age 6 from neurological complications.

The curve labeled "loss of milestones" represents children with diseases in which the loss of milestones begins later in life than in Tay-Sachs disease. Here, intellectual development is reasonably normal until 4–6 years of age, when neurological functions deteriorate and milestones are lost. The neurological functions of these children will continue to deteriorate throughout their lives.

The developmental pattern of a particular child provides important information that doctors use to focus their evaluations. Each abnormal developmental pattern suggests a particular category of diseases that require different diagnostic tests. A child with mental retardation will require a different set of tests than a child with loss of developmental milestones.

Now that we have defined the terms used to describe mentally handicapped children, we can begin to identify some causes of these handicaps.

Chapter 3

Nature, Nurture, and Genetics

There are many possible causes of mental disability. The disability may be mental retardation, learning disability, developmental delay, mental illness, or emotional disorder. In order to understand how factors contribute to or determine the handicap of any child, we must consider the interaction of two forces that influence human behavior—nature and nurture.

Nature can be defined as unchangeable physical attributes of an individual. This term includes genetic factors and predetermined instinctual behavior patterns. Nature also includes permanent physical disability as the result of accidents or infections. These forces will remain constant throughout the lifetime of an individual.

Nurture can be defined as those changeable external forces that act upon an individual. Individuals are influenced by their parents, other family members, teachers, peers, and their environment.

Sometimes the impact of nature-caused disability can be mediated by appropriate nurture. For example, the handicap of a child with congenital deafness (deafness since birth) can be decreased by teaching the child sign language and lip-reading. Failure to recognize deafness and to initiate appropriate therapies can result in infantile autism (Minshew & Payton, 1988a,b; see Chapter 13). A unified approach to an individual with a mental handicap must take into account both physical, nature-caused factors and nurture-caused factors.

Such an integrated approach to children with mental handicaps is a recent development. As recently as 10 years ago, it was assumed that the prognosis for children with Down syndrome was dismal and unalterable. Down syndrome, formerly called mongolism or mongolian idiocy, is a genetic disease causing peculiarly shaped faces, mental retardation, and other abnormalities. Children with Down syndrome were either placed in custodial institutions or kept sheltered at home. Children with Down syndrome who received no special remediation did poorly. We now know that appropriate interventions can dramatically improve the outcome for children born with Down syndrome. Infant stimulation programs (see Chapter 12) help children develop skills at a faster rate. Prompt medical intervention for problems especially associated with Down syndrome also improves functioning. For example, many children with Down syndrome suffer from hearing loss. This prevents them from developing normal speech patterns. Recognition of this problem and the provision of hearing aids can prevent speech disability. Infant stimulation programs and physical therapy can improve motor skills. Dental and orthopedic problems, frequent in children with Down syndrome, can be treated, and prompt recognition and treatment of these problems improve physical appearance and social acceptability. With optimum medical, emotional, educational, and therapeutic support, many individuals with Down syndrome are now able to hold semi-skilled jobs and live in supervised housing.

It is usually a combination of nature and nurture that eventually determines the outcome for any child with a mental handicap. It is always important to identify the etiology of a child's handicap, if at all possible, in order to provide the appropriate interventions (nurture) to alleviate nature-caused handicaps.

Nature or Nurture?

Few human traits can be attributed solely to nature or nurture. Even physical (nature) traits can be modified. Few people would dispute the statement that eye color is nature-caused: eye color is determined solely by an individual's genetic makeup. However, even such a simple trait can become complicated. An individual with brown eyes who chooses to wear blue contact lenses succeeds in disguising his natural eye color. What color are his eyes? Purists argue that his eyes are brown; others argue that the *appearance* of his eye color is now a nurture-caused trait because he can change it at will.

Hair color is another example of a physical trait in which nature and nurture combine to create the final result. Genetic factors determine the basic hair color of an individual, but exposure to sunlight will lighten some people's hair, and dyes and tints will obviously change its color. The final hair color of an individual is determined by a *combination* of the natural (genetic hair color) and the nurtural (sunlight exposure, and hair dyes). The contribution of each element to the final hair color will vary from individual to individual.

The same *physical* handicap may be caused by 100% nature, 100% nurture, or a combination of these factors. Blindness is a good example of such a phenomenon. I am often asked, "Is blindness genetic?" or "I have a son who is blind since birth, what are the chances I will have another blind child?" or "I have been blind since birth, what are the chances that my children will be blind?" I cannot answer accurately until I discover the original cause of the blindness.

Blindness can have a genetic cause. In the genetic disease Leber's congenital amaurosis, blindness is caused when a child inherits defective genes from both his parents. This is 100% nature. On the other hand, blindness may be caused completely by nurture in cases of hysterical blindness following severe emotional trauma.

Another possibility is that blindness may be caused by a combination of both nature and nurture. A good example of this is a disease called familial retinoblastoma. In order for an individual to suffer from familial retinoblastoma, he or she must possess a single abnormal gene. However, this gene is not sufficient to cause blindness. Individuals who have inherited this defective gene from one of their parents have an 80% risk of developing cancer in both eyes in infancy, causing blindness. This means that 20% of all people who have inherited this bad gene will not develop the eye tumors.

I care for Mary, a girl whose mother's brother and father became blind as a result of the eye tumors. Mary's mother had no tumors in her eyes, but Mary and her brother both developed tumors in early infancy. Mary's mother carries a defective gene (that she inherited from her father) and she passed it down to both her children. Mary's mother happens to be one of the fortunate 20% of individuals who carry the defective gene but do not develop tumors. The defective gene is not, in and of itself, sufficient to cause the development of eye tumors. Something else must occur (nurture), possibly a toxic environmental exposure or an infection, to cause the eye tumors to grow. Nature (the defective gene) and nurture (the second exposure) *combine* to cause blindness in familial retinoblastoma. Since 80% of people with the defective gene will eventually develop tumors, we can estimate that in this disease, nature contributes to 80% of the trait (blindness) and nurture contributes 20%.

Untreated eye infections are the most common cause of blindness in developing countries. Appropriate nurture (treatment of the infections) can completely prevent the blindness so in these cases the blindness is caused 100% by nurture.

Blindness can be caused by several different factors which represent various combinations of nature and nurture. Eye infections cause blindness and are not inherited; familial retinoblastoma is a genetic disease which, in combination with the environment, can cause blindness; and Leber's congenital amaurosis is a genetic disease that always causes blindness (Emery & Rimoin, 1983).

Since determining the etiology of such a "simple" trait as blindness is so difficult to sort out, imagine the complexity of trying to find the causes of mental retardation, mental illness, or behavioral problems! Although there are a few rare genetic diseases that cause predictable behavioral abnormalities 100% of the time (see Chapter 8), these are the exceptions and not the rules. They represent interesting examples of completely genetically (na-

ture) caused behavioral disorders, but one should not gen-
eralize from those few diseases and conclude that all mental handicaps are primarily caused by physical or genetic
problems.

Nature and Nurture: A Comment on Parenting

Parenting is not a one-way street. Even newborn babies have skills that endear them to their mothers, fathers,
and other adults. Most newborn infants cuddle their bodies into their parents, make eye contact with their parents,
and become calm when they hear voices or are gently
rocked. After a few months infants begin to smile in reflex
to their parents' smiles, and respond to the parents'
babytalk and efforts to soothe them. All these skills encourage parents to bond to their babies. For various reasons, some children do not have some or all of these
abilities. It is much more difficult to parent such a child.
It is much harder to bond to an infant who stiffens and
cries while being held or is unable, for whatever reason,
to respond to the usual parental cues. It may be very difficult for a parent to remain attached to a child who fails
to respond, and who actively resists cuddling and holding.
This phenomenon led to the erroneous conclusion that
parents of autistic children were at fault for the child's
malady because they were "refrigerator parents" (see
Chapter 2). Actually, autistic children reject parental contact.

Sometimes a child who is physically ill or mentally
handicapped is unable to respond in the usual ways to
parental caretaking. By the time the child is evaluated pro-

fessionally, the parents may be observed to have poor parenting skills or to interact "inappropriately" with their child. The tendency is for the professional to attribute any emotional disturbances in the child to poor parenting, when, in fact, the "poor parenting" and the emotional handicap may be the result of the child's neurological handicap and not the cause. It may be difficult to sort out whether ineffective parenting has caused emotional handicap or whether the child's physical or mental handicap has caused the "poor parenting."

I always give parents the benefit of the doubt and perform a full medical and genetic evaluation to see whether I can detect a physical cause for a problem in a child with developmental or emotional problems.

For example, I saw a 6-week-old baby and her mother in consultation. The mother had adopted this baby in the newborn period. She told me that the baby cried continuously, arched his back and stiffened up when held, and spit up after almost every feeding. She was tearful when she told me that it seemed that the baby didn't love her, and that she was becoming depressed and had thought of suicide. She told me, "I must be a terrible mother." Her baby had all the symptoms of an infant of a narcotics-addicted mother. These babies experience withdrawal symptoms after birth. We eventually learned that the biological mother of this baby was a heroin addict. I placed the baby on medication to alleviate some of the symptoms, and the adoptive mother learned about the care of addicted infants. This mother fared much better after she knew that her baby's suffering was not her fault and that the baby's behavior did not reflect upon her skills as a mother.

Since children of addicted mothers often have mental

handicaps, I fear what might have happened if the diagnosis of drug addiction had not been made in this case. Would this mother-child relationship have broken down? If this child developed emotional problems later on in life, would they be attributed to "poor parenting"? Would the adoptive mother be blamed for the lack of bonding in the newborn period?

Almost every parent of a handicapped child I see feels guilty about somehow causing or contributing to the difficulties of their child regardless of whether there is an objective reason to feel guilty. I have also found that no matter how many times I reassure parents, the guilt remains. Parents often blame themselves for their child's genetic diseases when they had no way of knowing about or changing their own genetic makeup.

If a medical diagnosis can be established for your child, the cause of the problem may be uncovered. Even if no diagnosis can be reached, ask your doctor about any concerns you may have over possible causes of your child's disability. If you don't ask, you will not be able to receive the important answers.

I was caring for a child with the genetic disease called the Fragile X syndrome. After establishing the diagnosis I asked if either parent had any questions. The mother asked me if her fall from a ladder in the third month of pregnancy could have caused this problem. My answer was a resounding "Absolutely not!" She did not seem reassured by my answer. I asked if she believed what I had told her. She said, "In my brain I believe you, Dr. Strom, but in my heart I still feel responsible." I referred this couple to a psychiatrist colleague of mine for counseling. Unfortunately they did not go. Three months later, at our next visit, she told me that she was still feeling guilty.

I again encouraged them to see my colleague. This time they took my advice and have begun to make progress.

Feelings of guilt will not help you, will not help your child, and will not help your marriage. Even in the unusual event when there is an objective foundation for guilt, guilt is a completely unproductive emotion. You must get on with the task of obtaining the best possible outcome for your handicapped child. This book will help you achieve optimum care for your child; it is up to you to get optimum care for yourself. It won't help your child if your marriage and personal life crumble because you have provided for your child's needs at the expense of your own needs and those of your spouse. I encourage you and your spouse to get professional counseling from psychologists, psychiatrists, social workers, and/or clergy. Although the tendency is to try to tough it out, any parent of a handicapped child will benefit from good counseling.

Choosing a counselor for yourself is just as important as choosing a doctor for your child. Sometimes a particular counselor just will not be right for you, despite his or her reputation. If you do not feel that you are getting any benefit from your therapy, seek another referral.

Chapter 4

Learning Disabilities and Attention Deficit Disorder

Before beginning a discussion about learning disabilities, I want to dispel a common misconception regarding optometry and learning disabilities.

Many people mistakenly feel that reading problems and other learning disabilities are due to poor coordination of eye movements. Many optometrists inflict costly and time-consuming eye exercises and therapies on children in an attempt to treat learning disabilities and dyslexia (inability to read). There is absolutely no evidence that these treatments have *any* beneficial effect on these children. It is simply a waste of money, time, and effort.

This is *not* to say that treatments for crossed eyes, nearsightedness, farsightedness, and lazy eyes (amblyopia) are not warranted. These are medical conditions which require treatment. But these treatments will not affect a child's learning disability. Obviously, if a child needs glasses, this will impact on his or her ability to read, and

the appropriate glasses should be obtained. It is untrue
that prisms and/or eye exercises will alleviate learning disabilities.

Learning Disabilities, Excluding Attention Deficit Disorder

As mentioned in Chapter 1, a child with a learning
disability will have a normal IQ but will have difficulty
learning in a mainstream classroom (for a review of learning disabilities, see Cruikshank, 1979). The diagnosis of
a learning disability can only be made by educational testing (sometimes called learning disability testing). There
are some clues that a child may have a learning disability
such as letter inversions and reversals, but most children
will demonstrate these phenomena to some degree in the
first and second grades. For example, many children with
no learning problems will make some letters backwards,
or reverse letters in a word ("was" instead of "saw"). Your
child's teacher will be able to tell you if the number and
type of your child's reversals are more than would be expected for his or her age and may be indicative of a possible learning disability. Educational testing is required to
appropriately diagnose a learning disability in a child along
with an assessment of his social and adaptive skills (see
Chapter 1).

I use the term *primary* learning disability to describe
children who have a learning disability with *no known*
physical, genetic, psychological, and/or social causes.
These children have an unexplained problem with brain
function that interferes with normal intellectual functioning. Children with primary learning disabilities often have

Table 4. Causes of Secondary
Learning Disability

Unrecognized sensorial handicap
   Hearing impairment
   Vision impairment
Mild cerebral palsy
Metabolic (biochemical) disease
Genetic disease
Birth defect syndrome
Attention deficit disorder* (primary or
   secondary)
Emotional disorder*
Social disorder*
Pharmacologic (caused by medicine)

*These problems may be the *result* of learning
disability, as well as the cause of learning disability.

secondary psychological symptoms in reaction to their disability.

Attention deficit disorders, social problems, and emotional disorders can all be the *result* of a primary learning disability as well as the *cause* of a *secondary* learning disability. If the learning disability is due to an identifiable cause, I classify it as a secondary learning disability. Table 4 illustrates some common causes of secondary learning disability.

By definition, children with learning disabilities have normal intelligence. Because of this they are acutely aware of their handicap and their inability to achieve goals attained by their peers. They are usually devastated by the knowledge that they are continually disappointing the authority figures in their lives, namely parents and teachers. Children have limited coping resources available to them.

Many will begin "acting out" and become behavioral problems or class clowns. Others will be become sullen and introverted. Some children will somatize and have constant complaints of stomach pains or headaches. Others will fidget constantly in their seats and appear to have a short attention span.

Behavior problems, attention problems, or the somatic (physical) complaints usually occur prior to the recognition of the learning disability. It is important for parents, teachers, and physicians to be aware of the possibility of a learning disability in a child with somatic complaints or behavioral problems that suddenly emerge at the beginning of kindergarten or first grade.

As noted earlier, children with a learning disability often have an extremely poor self-image because of their awareness of their inability to perform up to the expectations of themselves, their peers, their parents, and their teachers. It is common for such children to become depressed, have problems falling asleep, and be listless during the day.

Many children develop elaborate techniques to cover up their disability. One of my patients with a biochemical genetic disease (the cause of his learning disability) became the class clown, and was continually making jokes and disrupting the class in attempts to deflect attention from his deficits. Other children become withdrawn in class, hoping never to be called upon to offer information. Others will ask repeatedly to go to the bathroom or go to the nurse's office so that they will miss certain classroom activities.

One cannot assume that the *cause* of a learning disability is an emotional, social, psychological problem, or even an attention deficit disorder, because all of these problems can be the result of the disability rather than the cause.

Every child deserves the benefit of a complete medical (genetic and/or neurological), educational, and psychological evaluation before attributing causality to an emotional problem, learning problem, or school problem. A child who appears to be hyperactive and have autistic tendencies may actually be hearing-impaired or have the genetic disease Fragile X syndrome (see Chapter 6).

Before appropriate therapy can be provided, an adequate diagnosis must be established. It does little good to begin psychological counseling alone for a boy who is acting out in first grade when his primary problem is dyslexia (inability to read). The appropriate intervention for this child is tutoring and alternative learning programs in *addition* to psychological counseling.

The diagnosis of a primary learning disability can only be made after physical causes have been eliminated and after the administration of an appropriate battery of tests. Vision and hearing testing, appropriate medical testing, genetic evaluations, and educational testing should be carried out as soon as a child is identified as having a potential learning disability. If there is a behavioral component to the child's problem, a psychological or psychiatric evaluation should be carried out as soon as possible. There is no way to prioritize these evaluations. All should be performed, because even if a child has a treatable medical cause for a learning disability, he or she will still need to have the disability defined and appropriate remediation designed by educational testing. Similarly, if a child with a biochemical problem is not diagnosed and treated, educational progress will continually be impeded.

Testing of children with learning disabilities may be called educational testing, learning disabilities testing, or psychological testing, depending on the training of the person administering the test. Such testing will involve the administration of different tests usually over several sessions. The exact tests administered will vary for each child as the examiner will choose the appropriate tests for the child's age and level of functioning. The school district or your pediatrician should be able to provide parents with the names of individuals who perform educational testing (see Sattler, 1988, for complete descriptions of testing methods).

Although the learning disabilities tests have been designed to provide an objective measurement of a child's functioning, the performance of any individual child can vary greatly, depending on many factors other than the child's innate abilities. The child's physical and emotional state on the day of testing, the skills of the examiner, the interaction between the child and the examiner, the testing environment, and other intangibles all can influence a child's performance. For example, if an examiner fails to interest the child or hold his attention, the child will score lower than if the child had been engaged. One of the most important parts of any report of educational testing is the introduction, when the examiner describes his or her impressions of the effort level of the child.

I am continually amazed at how some examiners are consistently able to engage a child and obtain accurate testing. Testing reports from such individuals are tremendously helpful in establishing a diagnosis and initiating a treatment plan. In such cases there is a congruence between the child I am examining and getting to know and the test results on my desk.

On the other hand, several times a year I will read a report, and then be surprised when I meet a child who is nothing at all like the child described in the report in front of me.

Sometimes the chemistry between a child and an examiner will just be wrong. Even the most skillful examiners will occasionally be confronted with a child whom he or she cannot engage. In such cases it is better to suspend the testing, and try again with another examiner or at another time.

If, as an educator or parent, you feel that test results do not accurately reflect the abilities (either strengths or weaknesses) of a child, it is of tremendous importance that these doubts be articulated and documented, so that new testing can be performed. I cannot stress too much how physicians, educators, and therapists rely on these test results to plan for the future of children. Poor testing can lead to an inappropriate treatment plan. Then the child is continually frustrated and will not progress.

Let's use the example of a child with poor vision. If the eye test is done poorly, a nearsighted child may be fitted with farsighted glasses. Although the glasses were purchased with hard-earned money and effort, and with the best of intentions, the child will refuse to wear the glasses, and if you force him to do so, he will become angry and frustrated. This is exactly what will happen if a child has had poor educational testing and an inappropriate treatment plan has been devised. If your child is not responding to a particular treatment plan, and is getting progressively harder to work with, the problem may be a poor treatment plan. The answer may lie in a new round of testing and a new treatment plan rather than giving up on the child.

So please, if there are *any* doubts regarding the validity of test results for a child, make sure that the record reflects your concern. Some children may be extremely difficult to test, but no child is impossible to test. It may take several days or weeks to obtain valid results, but the effort will have a tremendous impact on the quality of the child's future life and therefore must be done.

I will not focus on social, emotional, or psychological causes of learning disability because this is not my area of expertise. Certainly children who are having difficulty at school and have behavioral problems need an evaluation by a psychologist, psychiatrist, or social worker, and appropriate intervention and counseling. However, such children also require a full medical and genetic evaluation to make sure that there is no medical cause of their disability.

Attention Deficit Disorder

I think of a learning disability as a sign, whereas attention deficit disorder is a symptom. In medicine, a sign is an objective measurement, such as high blood pressure or a skin rash. Signs usually suggest a particular etiology or etiologies. Symptoms, however, are more subjective. These involve complaints, such as pain or shortness of breath. For example, a headache is a symptom, whereas a drooping eyelid is a sign that suggests the presence of migraine headaches.

In my experience, some children who are diagnosed as having an attention deficit disorder actually have a medical problem or a primary learning disability as the cause of their attention deficit disorder. The child's inability to sit still in class is often an attempt to distract peers and teachers from noticing his disability. (For a complete review of attention deficit disorder see Shaywitz and Shaywitz, 1987.)

Some children fidget continually in school but are able to concentrate on television or movies. Some children are unable to concentrate for more than five or ten minutes on anything. The second type of child has a higher probability of having a true attention deficit disorder than the first.

As with learning disabilities, I divide attention deficit disorder into two categories, *primary* (no other medical cause) and *secondary* (caused by an identifiable problem). (For an excellent review of attention deficit disorder, see Taylor, 1986.)

There are many genetic and medical problems that can result in a child being diagnosed as having attention deficit disorder. For example, most children with the genetic diseases Tourette's syndrome and Fragile X syndrome (see Chapter 8) are diagnosed as having attention deficit disorder. In addition, children with primary learning disability often have attention deficit disorder as a result of learning disability and not because of a primary problem with attention span.

Children with primary attention deficit disorder can have attention deficit disorder alone or in combination with excessive movements (hyperactive, hyperkinetic). Often children with attention deficit disorder with a hyperactive component become disruptive to the classroom.

For all intents and purposes, the terms hyperkinetic and hyperactive are synonymous. The definition of hyperactive or hyperkinetic is subjective. A good definition of a hyperactive child is a child whose movements are con-

Table 5. Causes of Secondary
Attention Deficit Disorder

Metabolic disease
Learning disability (primary or
    secondary)
Genetic disease
Birth defect syndrome
Cerebral palsy

sidered by his parents or teachers to be excessive. The same child may be considered hyperactive by one teacher in one classroom but not by a different teacher in a different classroom.

This variability is due to two causes. Firstly, the symptoms of children with attention deficit disorder and hyperactivity can vary greatly according to their comfort and anxiety level in a given situation. A particular teacher, or a particular combination of children may allow a hyperactive child to behave in a more controlled fashion than another. Secondly, different teachers may have different tolerances for disruptive behavior in their classroom.

In preschool children the term attention deficit disorder is usually used to describe children who seem to be constantly in motion, and who have difficulty settling down or concentrating tasks.

Boys with attention deficit disorder and hyperactivity are more likely to have aggressive behavior and therefore come to the attention of teachers at earlier ages than girls with the same problem. Causes of secondary attention deficit disorder are listed in Table 5 and include primary learning disability.

By examining Tables 4 and 5 in detail we can see a what appears to be a circular problem; learning disability can cause attention deficit disorder and attention deficit disorder can cause learning disability. In addition, emotional problems can cause both attention deficit disorder and learning disability, and can, in turn, be caused by attention deficit disorder and learning disability.

It is crucial to remember that the description of a child as having a learning disability or attention deficit disorder does not constitute a medical diagnosis. If your child is diagnosed as having an attention deficit disorder, he or she should have a complete neurological and genetic evaluation. Medical, psychological, and educational testing may point to one cause or another. However, after a complete evaluation, it may still be impossible to determine the primary cause of the problems.

The treatment for children with primary attention deficit disorder is very different than for children with primary learning disability. The therapy for attention deficit disorder is stimulant medication, whereas the therapy for learning disabilities is tutoring, physical and occupational therapy, and remediation.

If a child has an attention deficit disorder as part of his or her problems, and no cause of the attention problem can be identified, it is appropriate to begin a trial of stimulant medication.

Stimulant Medication in Attention Deficit Disorder

It is clear that stimulant medication has a tremendous benefit for some children with attention deficit disorder.

There are three commonly used stimulant medications used for the treatment of children with attention deficit disorder. These are Ritalin (methylphenidate), Dexedrine (dextroamphetamine), and Cylert (pemoline). All these drugs are closely related to each other, but, for reasons that are not clear, children often respond differently to each of the three medications.

In my experience, when the stimulant medications are effective for a child, the results are usually immediate, and dramatic. Like all medications, there are benefits and side effects to the stimulant medications. In children who have an excellent response to the stimulants, the benefits are so great that the side effects are easily tolerated. For children who have only a subtle beneficial response or no response to the medications, it will be up to the child, parents, and physician together to decide whether to continue the medication.

Stimulant drugs can have unpleasant side effects, especially sleep disorders and physical incoordination. If a child is deriving no benefit from the drug, he or she should not be receiving it. However, it is clear that some children (in my experience about one-third of children with attention deficit disorder) can derive significant benefit from the stimulant drugs. If attention deficit disorder has been diagnosed and stimulant medication prescribed, fill the prescriptions and give the drug a try. There are no known permanent side effects to stimulant medications. Since no permanent damage can occur by trying the drug there is no reason not to try stimulant medications under a doctor's supervision.

One of my patients is a high school student who has been on Ritalin for 10 years. He learned to adjust his medication schedule according to his needs. The Ritalin helped him concentrate on intellectual tasks but caused him to have less physical coordination. If he has an examination or difficult assignment he takes Ritalin to help him concentrate, but if he has a baseball game in the afternoon he skips his dose.

When stimulant medications work for a child, they usually do so immediately. Parents and the child notice the difference within hours of the first dose of the drug. I usually start a child on a low dose of stimulant. If the parents notice no change after a week, I increase the dose, and then if there is no effect, I discontinue the drug. If there has been a partial response, I may try a different stimulant medication.

Stimulant medications have received a lot of negative publicity. Like any other medications, stimulant medications have benefits and side effects. Since some children with attention deficit disorder derive significant benefit from taking the drug, fear of the side effects should not deter parents from beginning a trial of stimulant medications for a child with attention deficit disorder. Side effects of stimulant medications are reversible when the drug is discontinued.

Children with attention deficit disorder who have the genetic disease Tourette's syndrome may have a particular adverse reaction to the introduction of stimulant medication. Sometimes the stimulant will "unmask" Tourette's syndrome and the child will begin to have a bizarre behavior known as vocal tics (see Chapter 8). However, it is important to note that the medication did not *cause* the Tourette's syndrome, it simply unmasked the Tourette's syndrome. Children with Tourette's syndrome can benefit from stimulant medication but it usually must be given in combination with other drugs such as Haldol (haloperidol) to control the tics.

I saw an 8-year-old child whose parents were completely at the end of their rope. At age 4 the boy had been diagnosed as having an attention deficit disorder and Dexedrine was prescribed. The Dexedrine completely changed this boy's life. He was able to go to school successfully and interact well with his parents. Then, at age 6, while on vacation, the boy became agitated. His parents increased his dose of Dexedrine in an attempt to calm him down. The following morning the child awoke and began barking like a dog. At that time, they called their pediatrician, who took the child off the Dexedrine, and the attention deficit disorder returned with a vengeance.

In this case the child's attention deficit disorder was due to Tourette's syndrome. The barking is a symptom of Tourette's syndrome known as a vocal tic. The overdose of Dexedrine had unmasked the Tourette's syndrome, but did not cause it.

Although stimulant medications can unmask Tourette's syndrome, there is no reason to withhold them from affected children. Stimulants, either alone or in combination with the medication Haldol, to prevent the tics, can be extremely beneficial for children with Tourette's syndrome (Comings, 1986).

I placed this child on a moderate dose of Ritalin, and he has done much better, with no recurrence of the vocal tics. If tics develop or he continues to have trouble, Haldol can be added to the Ritalin.

Chapter 5

Nongenetic Causes of Mental Dysfunction

Understanding the cause of mental dysfunction in children is like peeling off the layers of an onion. Each discovery brings us a little closer to the center, but many of the secrets remain unexplained.

This chapter discusses known *nongenetic* causes of mental dysfunction. If any of these causes is present in a child's medical history, this is likely to be the explanation for his or her handicap; but rarely a child will have more than one problem contributing to his or her dysfunction.

A child with a mental disability requires a complete medical evaluation including a family history, social history, and a physical examination to discover any evidence of known causes of mental dysfunction. This process may result in a diagnosis or may lead to specific testing aimed at finding the cause and the treatment of the handicap. Sometimes, when I examine a child and take a medical history, an explanation for his or her handicap will be immediately apparent. Some disorders are easy to diagnose but others may be impossible to confirm. When a diagnosis cannot be confirmed with reasonable certainty, the child is considered to have "unexplained" disability.

The next nine sections identify known nongenetic causes for mental dysfunction.

Prenatal Damage (Birth Defects)

Many agents are capable of injuring an unborn baby before birth. These agents are collectively known as *teratogens*. This word comes from the Greek words for "monster" and "forming." The effects of a teratogen may be recognized at birth if there is a physical defect or a severe mental handicap. The flipperlike arms and legs of babies exposed to the medication thalidomide and the blindness and skin rash caused by prenatal infection with the rubella virus (German measles) are examples of such obvious prenatal damage.

Many teratogens, however, have much more subtle effects that may not be noticeable at birth. Sometimes months or even years pass before the damage is recognized. For example, prenatal infection with the parasite Toxoplasma can lead to subtle visual impairment and/or learning disabilities that may not be detected until school age. A pregnant woman may have no noticeable symptoms from toxoplasma infection or just have nonspecific flu-like symptoms. Since the diagnosis of congenital infection with toxoplasmosis can only be confirmed in the newborn period, it is impossible to make a diagnosis in a school-aged child. Therefore, many children who have suffered brain

Table 6. Agents Capable of Causing Mental Dysfunction by Prenatal
Exposure

Infections*
  Rubella (German measles)
  Varicella (chickenpox)
  Cytomegalovirus (CMV)
  Herpes simplex (herpes)
  Human Immunodeficiency Virus Type 1
    (HIV1 - AIDS virus)
  Syphilis
  Toxoplasmosis
Environmental agents
  Lead
  Mercury
Alcohol (regular use)
Illegal drugs (cocaine, heroin, metha-
    done, etc.)
Prescription drugs
  Cancer chemotherapy
  Acutane (an acne medication)
  Thyroid medication

*Modified from Strom (1988).

damage from prenatal exposure to damaging agents will
remain undiagnosed. A list of teratogens capable of causing mental disability appears in Table 6. (For a complete
discussion of teratogenic agents please refer to Strom,
1988.)

    Any mentally handicapped child with a history of pre-
natal exposure to alcohol, lead (paint scrapings), insecticides, herbicides, or vitamin A preparations may have
suffered prenatal brain damage and should be evaluated
by a geneticist.

It is difficult to know whether or not a mother con-
tracted an infection with one of the harmful agents during
pregnancy because most of them cause only mild, nonspecific symptoms. A baby can be tested, however, in the
newborn period. So if there is any question that an infant
may have a birth defect or mental handicap, have him or
her evaluated immediately.

In *Have a Healthy Baby* (Strom, 1988), I tell pro-
spective parents how to protect their unborn babies from
prenatal damage.

Prematurity with Complication

Babies who are born prematurely (more than 4 weeks
before their due date) are often unable to survive without
intensive medical support. These "premies" are cared for
in special medical units called "NICU's" or "ICN's" (*Neo-*
natal *I*ntensive *C*are *U*nits or *I*ntensive *C*are *N*urseries).

Prematurity, in and of itself, does not cause brain
damage, but complications of prematurity can result in
brain damage. The medical problems of premature babies
are quite variable, depending on differences in the size
and gestational age (length of the pregnancy) of the infant.
Babies born as many 15 weeks before the due date (gestational age of 25 weeks) and weighing as little as one
pound have survived and gone home healthy, but, in general, larger babies and babies born closer to their due date
usually have fewer complications and subsequent handicaps
than these tiny premies.

A history of prematurity is not a sufficient explanation
for a mental handicap in a child. The following is a list

of key questions for parents to ask their doctors regarding the history of a premature baby. If the answer to any of these questions is yes, then there is a increased risk that the baby suffered brain damage. Medical terminology is given in parentheses.

1. Was the birth weight of the baby less than 1500 grams (3 lbs 4 oz.) (very low birth weight)?
2. Was the baby born more than 8 weeks early (32 weeks gestation)?
3. Was the baby on a breathing machine (ventilator) for more than 1 week?
4. Did the baby experience bleeding in the brain (intraventricular hemorrhage)?
5. Did the baby have epileptic convulsions (seizures) and require epilepsy medicine (anti-convulsant medication) while in the nursery?
6. Did the baby have any proven major infections (sepsis, meningitis, pneumonia)?
7. Did the baby have water on the brain (hydro-cephalus)?

Children who have suffered from one or more of these problems should be observed closely for any signs of mental dysfunction.

Birth Injury

A baby can suffer brain damage during labor and delivery if the brain is deprived of oxygen for prolonged periods. This is called perinatal asphyxia. The two most reliable predictors of perinatal asphyxia are the baby's Apgar scores and a history of seizures (epileptic convulsions) in the newborn period. Apgar scoring was developed to evaluate the condition of newborn infants. The Apgar evaluation examines 5 crucial factors in a newborn baby: heart beat, breathing, color, muscle tone, and reflexes. Each factor is given a score of 0, 1, or 2. A "perfect" score is 10. The worst possible score is 0. The Apgar evaluation is performed twice, first at 1 minute after birth and then at 5 minutes after birth. The results of these examinations are called the 1-minute and 5-minute Apgar scores respectively. In general, a 5-minute Apgar score of 8–10 means that the child has not suffered from significant lack of oxygen during the birth process. A 5-minute Apgar score of 3 or less indicates that the baby has had significant oxygen deprivation and may have suffered brain damage as a result.

The key questions to ask about the birth process are:

1. What were the Apgar scores of the baby?

2. How long did the baby have to stay in the nursery before he or she came home? (If a baby is hospitalized longer than the mother, this suggests a medical complication.)

3. Did the baby have any convulsions (epileptic seizures) in the newborn period? Seizures in the newborn period usually indicate brain damage suffered either prenatally or during birth.

4. Did the baby require any intravenous medicine or intramuscular medicine (shots) after birth? Babies with infections require antibiotic treatment.

5. Did the baby require intravenous fluids or require

tube feedings in the newborn period? Newborns who suffered brain damage will often be neurologically depressed
and may be unable to feed properly.

If the baby had Apgar scores over 3 and went home
with his mother and did not require any medication, then
there is probably no need to be concerned about perinatal
brain damage.

Perinatal Infection

The immune system of newborn infants is vulnerable.
Newborn infants under the age of 6 weeks are susceptible
to overwhelming infections that may cause only minor
illnesses in older children. Chicken pox and Herpes viruses
can cause significant brain damage and even death in newborn babies. The immune systems of newborn babies are
unable to prevent infections from spreading to the brain
from other parts of the body. Therefore newborns who
have pneumonia or other major infections may suffer brain
damage from the spread of the infection into the brain.
Until 6 weeks of age, an infection of any part of the body
has the potential to cause brain damage. After that time,
only specific infections of the brain will cause brain damage.

So, if a child has had one of the following infections
before the age of six weeks, this is likely to be the explanation for any subsequent mental dysfunction.

1. Generalized infection (sepsis)
2. Chicken pox
3. Herpes

4.   Pneumonia
5.   Meningitis
6.   Encephalitis
7.   Urinary tract infection (pyelonephritis)
8.   AIDS

After 6 weeks of age meningitis and encephalitis (infections of the brain and surrounding structures) may cause brain damage. Such brain damage may be subtle and unnoticeable until several years after the infection, when intellectual impairment may be noted. Many children will have hearing loss as a result of meningitis.

Preventable Causes of Mental Dysfunction

Kernicterus

Kernicterus causes brain damage because a substance called bilirubin poisons brain cells. Bilirubin is a yellow chemical that is a breakdown product of hemoglobin, the main component of red blood cells. Accumulation of bilirubin in the blood occurs to some extent in all newborns, causing their skin to turn yellow (jaundice). Kernicterus can be prevented by making sure that the bilirubin levels in the blood do not become dangerously elevated, but once elevations exceed the critical range, irreversible brain damage occurs.

Therefore, blood bilirubin levels are monitored religiously in hospital nurseries. When a baby's bilirubin levels become mildly elevated, he is often placed under fluorescent lights (bilirubin lights) to help his body get rid of the extra bilirubin. If his levels become dangerously elevated, the baby can be given an exchange transfusion, a process in which all his blood is replaced with donor blood.

Surveillance and treatment of bilirubin elevations is so strict in the United States that kernicterus has been virtually eliminated. If a child was not born in a hospital or was born in an underdeveloped country, kernicterus might be a possible cause of mental dysfunction. For a baby born in a hospital in the United States, a history of jaundice does not indicate a risk of brain damage unless the bilirubin levels were dangerously elevated.

Congenital Hypothyroidism

Children who are born without functional thyroid glands will, if not treated immediately with replacement thyroid hormone, become mentally retarded, and dwarfed. The medical term for such children is Cretin. In the United States, Canada, and Western Europe, newborn screening programs check all newborns for congenital hypothyroidism. However, some children with congenital hypothyroidism can be missed. Not all children are screened, and screening tests do not pick up all of the forms of congenital hypothyroidism. If a child has poor growth and developmental delay, a medical evaluation is needed to check for this disease.

The diagnosis of congenital hypothyroidism is crucial because treatment with replacement thyroid hormones completely prevents the mental handicap and growth abnormalities.

Brain Injury

There are many causes of brain injury. Shock, head trauma and child abuse, near drowning, choking, stroke, open heart surgery, and low blood sugar can cause brain injury. Cerebral palsy is a condition that results from brain damage, but the cause of the damage is usually unknown.

Shock

Shock is the inability of the body to circulate enough blood to keep the vital organs (including the brain) supplied with sufficient oxygen to prevent damage. Shock can cause brain injury. Dehydration from diarrhea and vomiting, major infections, ruptured appendixes, accidents (trauma), and chemical imbalances may cause shock. Any child with a history of these problems may have suffered from shock. Subsequent mental disabilities may be the result of an episode of shock.

Head Trauma and Child Abuse

Children who have had significant trauma to the head as the result of an accident or as the result of child abuse can suffer brain injury. "Shaken child syndrome" describes a form of child abuse in which brain injury is sustained as a result of a child being shaken. Careful physical examination of the back of the eye, and computerized X rays of the brain are necessary to establish this diagnosis; there may be no obvious external indications of trauma.

It is not known how many children suffer undetected brain injury from being shaken.

Near-Drowning or Choking

Children who survive being submerged in water for more than five minutes or choking on food for similar periods of time usually sustain brain injury resulting from a lack of oxygen to the brain. If the lack of oxygen is severe enough to cause significant brain injury, the child will be sick enough to require hospitalization following the episode. There is no reason to suspect brain injury in a child who was evaluated in an emergency room and immediately released following one of these episodes.

Children who have been trapped in fires can have brain injury secondary to carbon monoxide poisoning or inhaling other toxic substances. If enough damage has occurred to cause brain injury the child will require hospitalization.

Stroke and Open Heart Surgery

Children who require open heart surgery to repair heart defects must be placed on a heart-lung machine. This procedure places them at risk for having brain injury caused by a blood clot blocking a blood vessel in the brain (stroke). Some heart defects can allow blood clots to travel to the brain, causing damage.

There is one particular genetic disease called homocystinuria that can cause strokes in children. This is discussed in Chapter 9.

Hypoglycemia

Hypoglycemia occurs when an individual's blood sugar level becomes too low. Prolonged fasting, insulin overdose, and certain biochemical abnormalities (discussed in Chapter 9) are capable of causing hypoglycemia. The symptoms of hypoglycemia include seizures, cold clammy skin, racing heart beat, nausea, and light-headedness.

Hypoglycemia can be caused by insulin overdose in children with diabetes receiving insulin injections. Infants can also suffer from recurrent hypoglycemia and usually will have seizures as the result of the blood sugar becoming too low. Low blood sugar can cause brain damage by starving the brain of its primary nutrient. Several inborn errors of metabolism capable of causing recurrent hypoglycemia are discussed in Chapter 10.

Cerebral Palsy

The brains of children with cerebral palsy (C.P.) malfunction in particular ways. In most cases of cerebral palsy the child has a structurally normal brain that somehow sustained permanent damage. Although some cases of cerebral palsy are clearly caused by brain damage during the birth process, in most cases the cause is not known. For many years poor obstetrical practice was blamed for causing all cases of cerebral palsy, but recent studies have shown that most children with cerebral palsy had normal Apgar scores and did not show other signs of deprivation of oxygen during labor and delivery.

Children with cerebral palsy have different symptoms depending on the part of the brain that has been injured.

They usually have normal intelligence, but intellectual handicap (learning disabilities or mental retardation) may accompany cerebral palsy. Although severe cases of cerebral palsy are easy to diagnose, many children are only mildly affected. Sometimes the first indication of mild cerebral palsy is that a child walks on his or her toes. This can be due to spastic contractions of the calf muscles. One particular form of cerebral palsy results in abnormal movements and posturing (called chorio-athetosis). If you observe a child with definite movement problems or abnormal writhing or posturing movements, a referral to a pediatric neurologist should be made to evaluate the possibility of cerebral palsy.

It is important to note that although the brain damage in cerebral palsy is thought to have occurred before birth, many children with mild cerebral palsy will not have recognizable symptoms at birth. It may take several months or even years for the symptoms of cerebral palsy to become noticeable in a child.

Hydrocephalus (Water on the Brain)

Inside the brain are reservoirs of fluid called ventricles. Like lakes, the ventricles have inlets where fluid is created and outlets where fluid is resorbed. If the outlet to the ventricles is blocked, fluid will accumulate in the ventricles and the ventricles will expand and put pressure on the brain. This can cause brain injury. Hydrocephalus can be caused by many different mechanisms. Congenital hydrocephalus (present at birth) can be caused by genetic problems or by prenatal infection. Hydrocephalus can develop in a premature baby if intraventricular hemorrhage (bleeding into the brain) occurs. Children who survive brain infections (meningitis, tuberculosis meningitis, or encephalitis) can develop hydrocephalus.

Regardless of the cause of hydrocephalus, it is treated in the same way. A plastic tube is placed into the ventricles and the tube is threaded under the skin and emptied into the abdominal cavity. This procedure is called a shunt. Shunts can become infected or can malfunction. Children with hydrocephalus who have shunts in place may have residual brain damage caused either by the hydrocephalus itself or by complications of the shunt placement, shunt malfunction, or shunt infections.

Seizures (Convulsions, Epilepsy)

Seizures do not usually cause brain damage. However, in infancy, seizures may be a symptom of an underlying biochemical problem or brain injury or brain abnormality. Childhood epilepsy can be divided into three different categories.

Seizures in Infancy

This is the most ominous category of seizures with respect to future mental dysfunction. The seizures may begin in the newborn period or in the first few months of life and usually require anticonvulsant medication to control. The seizures may be dramatic, such as grand mal seizures, characterized by twitching of arms and legs, or may be more subtle, with a brief jerk or loss of consciousness. Petit mal seizures are benign and are discussed below.

Medical terms for the various types of non-grand mal or non-petit mal seizures are: minor motor seizures, infantile spasms, myoclonic jerks, myoclonic seizures, absence attacks, and salaam attacks. Although these seizures appear less frightening than grand mal seizures, they often indicate severe problems in the brain. A history of any one of these seizure disorders in infancy provides an explanation for subsequent mental dysfunction. Such children require close supervision by a pediatric neurologist.

Grand Mal Seizures Beginning in Children over 2 Years of Age

Sometimes children may have a single grand mal seizure associated with a high fever. This is called a simple febrile convulsion. It does not require any medication and has no future significance for the child's health or mental development. Other children can develop grand mal seizures that require anticonvulsant medication to control. Often these children outgrow their need for medication by adolescence. These children have no higher incidence of intellectual or mental dysfunction than children with no history of seizures. Therefore, the presence of this type of seizure disorder does not provide an explanation for mental handicap.

Petit Mal Seizures

Petit mal seizures are a particular form of benign seizure when a child suddenly "spaces out" for few seconds. Sometimes his eyes appear to glaze over or roll up in his head during a petit mal seizure, but this is not always the case. Children with petit mal seizures do not remember having them. They are totally unaware that anything has happened. The diagnosis of petit mal seizures is confirmed by a brain wave test (electroencephalogram, or EEG). These children have specific brain wave patterns during a seizure that can be captured by the EEG machine. A neurologist can induce a seizure by asking the child to breathe rapidly (hyperventilate). In children who cannot cooperate by hyperventilating, seizures can be induced by sleep deprivation (sleep-deprived EEG).

In any event, petit mal seizures are treatable with specific anticonvulsant medications and *do not cause brain injury or mental handicap*. Sometimes, however, if a child with petit mal seizures is not diagnosed and treated, the periods of "spacing out" can negatively affect his or her school performance. If you notice a child having episodes of "spacing out" for brief periods, a referral to a neurologist is necessary. It may be very difficult to determine if it is just daydreaming or petit mal seizures by simply observing the child. An EEG, however, can unequivocally establish the presence of petit mal epilepsy.

It is possible for the EEG to miss some cases of epilepsy. Sometimes, if the clinical suspicion is great enough, a child can be placed on seizure medication on a trial basis to see if his school performance improves with the therapy.

Toxic Exposure

The brains of infants and children are extremely vulnerable to damage by toxic metals, such as lead and mercury. Lead is contained in paint, leaded gasoline, and diesel fuel, and in soil near areas of congested vehicle traffic. Mercury is found in insecticides and herbicides. The symptoms of *acute exposure* (sudden large exposure) to lead include headache, nausea, vomiting, dizziness, unsteadiness, and seizures (epilepsy). Usually, however, lead exposure is chronic, occurring at low levels over a long period of time. The symptoms of chronic, low-level lead exposure are much more subtle. Clumsiness in fine motor coordination, inability to pay attention in school, and decreasing school performance may be the only signs of chronic lead exposure. Children are much more sensitive to the toxic effects of lead than are adults; children may be affected while their parents are totally asymptomatic from the same exposure. A blood test can determine if your child is suffering from lead poisoning.

When it was discovered that ingestion of lead by infants and toddlers could cause brain damage, lead was removed from most indoor painting products. Lead is still present in many exterior paints and in interior paints more than 20 years old. Lead is also found in pottery and ceramic products from Third World countries. Enough lead can be leached from ceramic pitchers, plates, and pots to cause lead poisoning.

Today lead poisoning is seen mainly in children from inner cities, where there is a lot of old, peeling paint. In addition, poor children are often nutritionally deprived and become iron-deficient. Iron deficiency can cause a phenomenon known as pica, when people eat large amounts of nonfood items such as dirt and paint chips. These are often contaminated with lead. Lead poisoning is also seen in children who are living in homes undergoing extensive remodeling involving paint scraping, furniture-stripping, and/or redecorating. Rarely, a child will become lead poisoned from the use of pottery or ceramic items made with lead containing glazes.

Children who live in farm areas can be affected by exposures to mercury compounds found in insecticides and fungicides. Infants and children are much more susceptible to brain injury from these toxic substances than adults. *Any child living on a farm who has mental dysfunction should be evaluated for possible toxic exposures.*

This chapter has acquainted you with nongenetic causes of mental handicap in children. If you feel your child may have suffered from any of these problems, consult your doctor for an appropriate evaluation or referral to diagnose these problems. If none of the above problems are present in a child, a complete genetic evaluation is warranted to evaluate for the possibility of a genetic disease or multiple malformation syndrome (Chapter 8).

Some parents ask me, "Just because my child has a nongenetic explanation for his dysfunction, couldn't he still have a genetic problem?" The answer to this question is that anything is possible. You may still wish to have a genetic evaluation of your child even though one of the other explanations is present. Ask your doctor or other specialist whether your child's symptoms are all explained by the causative agent you have discovered. If the answer is no, you may want to have your child evaluated by a geneticist.

What Examinations Will Your Baby Have before Leaving the Hospital?

After a baby is born in a hospital, certain routine tests and examinations are performed. It is important to understand what a normal newborn evaluation means, and the limitations of these tests. The fact that the results of these tests are all normal does not insure that your child will not develop a mental handicap.

The hospital staff performs certain tests and functions for all newborns. Initially, the nurses wash your baby, take his or her temperature, place antibiotic eyedrops in the eyes, and give an injection of vitamin K (Aquamephyton). The vitamin K prevents certain bleeding problems in newborns, and the antibiotic eye drops prevent the possibility of blinding eye infections.

If the nurses do not note any problems, your baby will be examined by a physician sometime in the first 24 hours of life and again prior to discharge. These examinations may be performed by a resident physician (a doctor-in-training) or by your designated pediatrician (attending physician). This first examination is called the admission newborn examination, and the second, the discharge examination. The physician will examine your baby carefully for physical birth defects. The heart, lungs, abdomen, genitals, spine, head, ears, hips, and eyes will all be examined for signs of defects.

There are two aspects to brain function. *Cortical function* (involving the *cerebral cortex*) is what we associate with intellectual functioning. These functions are controlled by the higher (cortical) centers of the brain. *Brain stem functioning* involves unconscious reflexes and the regulation of body functions such as temperature and heart rate. It is extremely difficult to assess cortical functioning in a newborn. The standard newborn physical examination primarily assesses brain stem functioning of a newborn baby. I have seen babies who "passed" their newborn physical examinations who had almost no brain at all.

Unfortunately, the fact that no abnormalities are observed on a routine newborn examinations is no assurance that your baby does not have a problem that may cause a mental handicap in the future.

There is a different sort of physical examination, called a Brazelton examination, a more sensitive measurement of cortical function than the routine newborn examination. Named after its pioneering founder, T. Berry Brazelton, the Brazelton examination tests some simple cortical functions in newborn infants such as cuddling, response to sounds and faces, and mood changes.

Performing a complete Brazelton examination requires patience and experience. The baby must be in an appropriate mood (the active alert, or quiet alert state) in order to perform an accurate Brazelton examination. Since pediatricians tend to come into the hospital at fixed periods of times, it is unlikely they will "catch" a baby at the right time. In addition, the Brazelton examination is time consuming to perform. Most pediatricians will attempt to assess some aspects of a Brazelton examination when examining newborns, but will rarely perform the entire examination prior to hospital discharge.

Although the Brazelton examination measures some aspects of cortical functioning, it provides only a rough estimate of total function. An abnormal Brazelton examination will alert the physician to the possibility of a future mental disability in a baby. However, a normal Brazelton examination does not insure that a child will develop no mental problems in the future. Feel free to ask your pediatrician about having a Brazelton examination performed on your infant. Often, an examiner will allow you to watch the examination and will point out your baby's skills.

Chapter 6

Mechanisms of Heredity

Before beginning our discussion of genetic diseases and inheritance we need to compare and contrast the terms *genetic* and *congenital*. These terms are not synonymous but are often, incorrectly, used interchangeably.

Congenital means existing from birth.

Genetic means caused by the hereditary elements (genes and chromosomes).

Not all *congenital* abnormalities are *genetic*. For example, by definition, congenital deafness is present at birth. However, congenital deafness can be caused by a variety of mechanisms. Infection in unborn babies can cause congenital deafness (congenital but *not* genetic). Many different genetic diseases can cause congenital deafness (congenital *and* genetic). Some genetic diseases cause progressive deafness so that the child is born with normal hearing and hearing loss begins several years later. In this case the deafness can be described as being *genetic*, but not congenital.

Since genetic diseases involve the hereditary elements, they are, by definition, present at birth. To be absolutely accurate, the diseases are actually present in the fertilized egg. However, some genetic diseases may not be *apparent* until well after birth. For example, infants with the genetic disease Tay-Sachs disease (see Chapter 9) appear completely normal at birth. It is only after mental deterioration is noticed, usually around 1 year of age, that this genetic disease causes symptoms. Tay-Sachs disease is an example of a disorder that *appears* to be genetic and not congenital but is actually both genetic and congenital.

This chapter addresses genetic issues. There are two categories of genetic diseases, those caused by an abnormal number or abnormal structure of cellular components called *chromosomes*, and those caused by defective *genes*. For an excellent basic review of human genetics see Thompson and Thompson (1986).

What Are Genes and Chromosomes?

All the information required to create an individual is present in the fertilized egg. The information is stored as a sequence of four different letters known as *bases*, strung together in a chemical chain known as DNA (deoxyribonucleic acid). Each base can be thought of as a different letter. The four letters are arranged in three-letter words called *codons*. There are only 22 different "words" in the genetic "dictionary." Twenty of the words correspond to the 20 different amino acids. These 20 amino acids are the building blocks of proteins. The two remaining words mean "start" and "stop." These words tell the cellular machinery when to begin reading the gene, and when to stop reading the gene. This collection of 22 three letter words is called "the genetic code."

A gene is a stretch of DNA that acts like a blueprint or a recipe to tell the cellular machinery how to make an individual protein. Each gene begins with the word start, continues with a string of three-letter words (codons) completely specifying the exact order of amino acids in the protein, and ends with the word stop. Some proteins are comprised of several hundred amino acids. Since there are 20 different amino acids that can be strung together in any order, there is a tremendous variety of proteins that can be specified by genes. The entire diversity of life on this planet is generated by variations in the sequence of genetic words specifying the structure of an almost infinite number of different proteins.

Each cell has machinery designed to read the words, just as an engineer can read a blueprint. The cellular machinery uses the gene as a blueprint and makes the various proteins according to the plan. The genetic code is the basis for all life on this planet. Even a microscopic yeast cell is capable of "reading" the most sophisticated gene in man.

In summary, a gene is a sequence of letters (bases) organized into three-letter words (codons) beginning with the word "start" and ending with the word "stop." The cellular machinery reads the gene and makes a protein by adding each block (amino acid) sequentially to the protein in the exact order specified by the gene. In this way genes specify the exact composition of a protein. For example, if a protein is supposed to be 100 amino acids long, then the gene will contain 300 bases arranged in order, forming 100 codons in between the "start" and "stop" codon.

There are about 100,000 genes in every cell in every

person. There are approximately 3 billion bases of DNA per cell in humans. The total length of DNA contained in each and every microscopic cell, if it were stretched into a straight line is estimated to be about 6 feet long! In order to fit that entire length of DNA into a cell, the DNA is wound around special proteins like thread wound around a spool.

Another way to think about the enormous amount of information stored in the DNA of every cell in your body is to compare it to books in libraries. Most books contain between 50,000 and 100,000 words on 150–250 pages. Since each word has an average of about 5 letters, each book has about 300,000 letters. Since the human genetic information is stored as 3 billion letters (3,000,000,000), the total amount of information stored in the DNA of every cell in our bodies would fill ten thousand (10,000) books. Each book would contain about 40 genes.

A single change in one of the 3 billion letters in the genetic sequence is called a *mutation*. A mutation is completely analogous to a single typographical error. It is mind-boggling that a single mutation is capable of causing lifelong suffering from a genetic disease.

In each cell, these 100,000 genes are strung end to end on 46 large chains of DNA called *chromosomes*. Using our library analogy, our 10,000 books will be organized on 46 different shelves with each shelf holding about 200 books. Each shelf would represent a different chromosome. In order to be completely analogous to a real chromosome, the books on each shelf would have to be combined into one giant book, because each chromosome contains only a single chain of DNA. Chromosomes vary in size. The largest chromosome, called chromosome 1, has about 6 inches of DNA and is about 5 times larger than the smallest chromosome, called chromosome 21. The normal human complement of chromosomes is 46. Forty-four of the 46 chromosomes occur in pairs and are called the *autosomes*. Thus there are 22 autosomal pairs. One of each pair of autosomes is inherited from the father and the other comes from the mother. The remaining 2 chromosomes are the sex chromosomes. One sex chromosome is inherited from each parent.

Each member of a pair of autosomal chromosomes contains the genes coding for the same proteins as its mate (*homologue*), so that everyone has 2 genes to code for each autosomal protein, one from the mother and the other from the father. There are approximately 2000–8000 genes on each chromosome.

The two chromosomes that are not autosomes are the *sex chromosomes*. The sex chromosomes comprise the 23rd pair of chromosomes. There are 2 types of sex chromosomes, X and Y. Each individual has one X chromosome and either a second X chromosome (females) or a single Y chromosome (males). Thus, if a baby inherits a single X chromosome from each of its parents it will be a girl, and if it receives an X chromosome from its mother and a Y chromosome from its father, it will be a boy. Since women do not have a Y chromosome, they can only give one of their X chromosomes to each of their children.

There are several hundred genes on the X chromosome that have various non-gender related functions. These are referred to as X-linked genes. As far as we can detect, however, there is only one functional gene on the Y chromosome, which is only active in the womb and causes the fetus to become a male.

The human Y chromosome is very interesting. Unlike all the other chromosomes which contain thousands of genes, scientists have only been able to identify one functional gene lying on the Y chromosome. Less than 1% of the total material on this chromosome actually functions as genetic material. The rest of the DNA is simply filler, which functions to insure that the Y chromosome lines up correctly during cell division. The actual size of the Y chromosome varies among different men. It is not the size of the Y chromosome that counts. All that is important is that the one gene comprising less than 1% of the total size of the chromosome, is present and is normal.

The one gene that is on the Y chromosome acts only once, after only a few weeks of embryonic life. The product of this gene causes testicles to develop in the embryo. In the absence of this material, the embryo will produce ovaries instead of testicles. Once the testicles are formed, they secrete male hormones responsible for making the baby into a male. Thus, in humans, maleness is the result of a positive action of the Y chromosome's gene, whereas femaleness is the result of the absence of this factor. There is no "female" factor that causes an embryo to develop as a girl. As far as we can tell, once the Y chromosome gene has induced the formation of testicles in very early embryonic life, it never functions again.

Therefore, there is an important distinction between men and women genetically. Women have two copies of all X-linked genes, whereas men have only one copy. I will explain in a later section how this puts men at increased risk for genetic diseases involving genes on the X chromosome.

What Is a Genetic Disease?

A genetic disease is caused by the presence of one or two abnormal genes out of the 100,000 genes comprising the genetic makeup of an individual. By definition, the cause of a genetic disease is the genetic makeup of the individual.

There are 1,906 proven genetic diseases listed in the most current compilation of genetic diseases, *Mendelian Inheritance in Man*, by Victor McKusick. There are three types of genetic diseases: *autosomal dominant, autosomal recessive*, and *X-linked*. Each one of these types of diseases has a characteristic pattern of inheritance. In an autosomal dominant disease, one parent has the disease and each of his or her children will have a 50% chance of inheriting the disease. In an autosomal recessive genetic disease, unaffected parents who carry the defective gene have a 25% risk of each of their children having the recessive disease. In X-linked diseases, if fathers have this disease, all their daughters will always be carriers of the disease. Their sons have a 50% chance of having the disease.

Single-Gene Disorders

A gene can be defined in general terms as the smallest unit of inheritance. Many traits such as color blindness or eye color are caused by the action of a single gene, whereas others are determined by the combination of the actions of several genes plus environmental factors.

Each individual has two copies of each autosomal gene. One copy is inherited from the mother (maternal) and the other is inherited from the father (paternal). If both inherited genes are identical, the individual is described as being *homozygous* for that gene, and the individual is called a *homozygote*. If the two genes are different, the individual is *heterozygous* for that gene and the individual is called a *heterozygote*. In genetic diseases, if a heterozygous individual is affected with the disease, the disease is called a *dominant disease*. In contrast, in a *recessive disease*, only individuals who have inherited two defective genes (one from each parent) can be affected. In such cases the parents who are heterozygous and have one good gene and one defective gene are called *carriers* for that particular genetic disease. Defective genes that cause diseases can be either recessive or dominant.

Autosomal-Dominant Diseases

The presence of a single defective gene causing a dominant genetic disease is sufficient to produce that disease in an individual. An example of this type of autosomal-dominant inheritance is Huntington's disease. Individuals afflicted with Huntington's disease appear completely normal until progressive mental deterioration begins between the ages of 30–50, eventually resulting in death. This disease is inherited as a dominant, therefore heterozygotes will have the disease. If one parent has a dominant genetic disease, then each child will have a 50% risk of inheriting the disease (heterozygous) and a 50% chance of being completely normal (homozygous normal).

Not all family members who have inherited the same dominant gene will be affected by the disease to the same degree. This phenomenon is termed *genetic variability* or *variable expression.* Sometimes a parent will have a very mild form of a dominant disease, but will have a child with a severe form of the same disease, even though their child inherited the *same* defective gene.

Neurofibromatosis is a dominant disease with variable expression and occurs with a frequency of 1 in 3300 births. The complete severe syndrome consists of multiple birthmarks called cafe-au-lait spots, multiple tumors of the skin, and multiple internal tumors involving the nerves. These tumors can cause deafness, blindness, mental retardation, and seizures. The "Elephant Man" had a form of neurofibromatosis. Another name for neurofibromatosis is von Recklinghausen's disease. Patients with the severe form of neurofibromatosis often die of malignant tumors at a young age.

The symptoms of neurofibromatosis have a wide variability even within the same family. Often a parent will have multiple birth marks called cafe-au-lait spots as the only indication that they have neurofibromatosis, but their child can be severely affected with the full syndrome, including both skin tumors and brain tumors. Other offspring may be moderately affected with birthmarks, skin tumors, seizures, mental retardation, or any combination of these problems.

A parent with a dominant disease has a 50% risk of passing the defective gene to each child, causing the child to have the disease. An unaffected individual does not possess the defective gene so is at no risk for having children with a dominant genetic disease.

Autosomal-dominant genetic diseases, including neurofibromatosis, often occur in children of parents who do not have the disease at all. This occurrence is referred to as *sporadic dominance.* Once the mutation has occurred, however, the affected individual will transmit the diseased gene to his offspring in the classic pattern of autosomal dominant inheritance. The parents, however, are at no increased risk of having a second child with the same mutation.

Therefore, because neither parent has a dominant genetic disease does not mean that the child cannot have the disease. Neurofibromatosis, Tuberous Sclerosis, and Marfan's Syndrome are examples of autosomal-dominant genetic diseases that can cause mental retardation and/or learning disabilities and are often present in children with unaffected parents.

The most frequent genetic cause of learning disabilities is a dominant defective gene (see Chapter 7). Families can have multiple generations affected with similar learning disabilities, with the abnormal gene being passed down from parent to child.

Autosomal-Recessive Diseases

In *autosomal-recessive genetic diseases*, only homozygotes that have two defective genes will be affected. By definition, heterozygotes will be unaffected. These unaffected heterozygotes are termed *carriers* of that particular genetic disease. Each individual with a recessive genetic disease must inherit one defective gene from each of his parents. Therefore each parent of a child with a recessive genetic disease *must* be a carrier of that disease. For some recessive genetic diseases, testing can determine if individuals are carriers prior to the birth of an affected child. This testing is recommended for members of certain ethnic groups with a high frequency of carriers for particular genetic diseases (for more details see my book *Have a Healthy Baby*). The risks for each child in a mating between two carriers of a recessive genetic disease are as follows:

> 25% will be affected with the disease (homozygous recessive)
> 50% will be carriers of the disease (heterozygous); and
> 25% will be normal (homozygous normal or homozygous dominant).

Genetic variability is also seen in recessive disorders. *Isovaleric acidemia* is an example of such a recessive genetic disease. Some children will be critically ill soon after birth, whereas others have recurrent episodes of vomiting associated with subtle deterioration of mental abilities as their only symptoms of the disease. This variability is even seen between two siblings who have inherited exactly the same defective genes from their parents (see Chapter 10).

Children with mild isovaleric acidemia may be totally asymptomatic until age 3–6 years, when they first begin having problems. Usually the first signs of difficulty are recurrent episodes of vomiting (without diarrhea). If unrecognized and left untreated, this disease can cause brain damage and can lead to mental retardation and/or learning disabilities. (For a more detailed discussion of isovaleric acidemia, see Chapter 8.) We do not yet understand all the contributing factors to genetic variability.

X-Linked Diseases

For *X-linked disorders*, the inheritance pattern is different than for autosomal diseases (either dominant or recessive). All males have only one X chromosome. This is described by the term *hemizygous*. Since women have two X chromosomes, the terms homozygous, heterozygous, and carrier still apply. Since all boys must inherit their Y chromosome from their fathers and an X chromosome from their mothers, all boys with X-linked genetic diseases must have a mother who is a carrier for that disease.

In contrast all girls must inherit their father's X chromosome. Thus, all daughters of a man with an X-linked disease will be carriers for that disease. The risks of X-linked genetic disease in offspring of a carrier female married to an unaffected male are:

daughters: 50% carriers (heterozygous)
50% normal (homozygous normal)
sons: 50% affected (hemizygous recessive)
50% normal (hemizygous normal)

Therefore, X-linked disease leads to distinctive family trees in which only males are affected, with transmission of the disease occurring through carrier females. A woman whose father has an X-linked disease must be a carrier, each of her sons will have a 50% risk of having the disease, and each of her daughters will have a 50% risk of being carriers. In addition, a woman who has a brother with an X-linked disease will have a 50% risk of being a carrier, because she had a 50% chance of inheriting her mother's defective gene.

If a disorder exhibits one of these three classical types of inheritance patterns, it is reasonable to assume that it is a genetic disease. However, mistakes can be made by using this logic. An interesting example of such a mistake occurred in the study of a fascinating disease called kuru in a cannibalistic tribe called the Fore of New Guinea. Kuru causes neurological deterioration and death within two years. The disease can begin anytime in life, but is always fatal. Many cases of kuru occurred within the same extended family, especially in children of affected parents. This led scientists to postulate that kuru is a dominantly inherited genetic disease. However, one fact cast doubt on this conclusion. *Wives* of affected men were also frequently affected, and there is no way for a man to give his genes to his wife. The resolution of this puzzle came with the isolation of a virus from the brains of individuals with kuru. The virus is responsible for the disease, and was spread in this tribe by the custom of cooking and eating the brains of deceased family members. If the loved one was infected with the virus his wife and children would contract kuru when they cooked and ate his brains. Kuru appeared to be genetic but it is actually an infectious disease. Since the tribe has refrained from eating the brains of individuals who have died of kuru, the disease has almost been eliminated from that population.

The example of kuru points out the problems inherent in jumping to conclusions about the genetic cause of any disease. Family members share many things other than their genes. Environmental exposures, infectious exposures, and parental exposure (i.e., parents who abuse their children) are also shared among siblings.

Chromosomal Diseases

Chromosomal diseases are caused by an abnormal amount (either too much or too little) of chromosomal material. The chromosomal content of any individual can be analyzed from samples of his skin, blood, or bone marrow. Analysis of the chromosomal content of any individual is called a *karyotype*. This type of analysis has been available for the past two decades.

The results of a karyotype are reported in the following way. The total number of chromosomes appear first, followed by a comma. Then the two sex chromosomes are listed. Thus a normal female karyotype is 46,XX and a normal male karyotype is 46,XY. If there are any abnormalities, these are listed after the sex chromosomes.

After birth, karyotyping can be performed on blood samples, bone marrow samples, or on skin cells that have been removed and grown in a test tube. Karyotypes can also be performed on unborn babies' cells obtained by a technique called *amniocentesis* or by analyzing fetal cells in the placenta using a procedure known as *chorionic villus sampling* (CVS).

Down Syndrome

The most common genetic disease in the general population is *Down syndrome* (formerly known as mongolian idiocy, or mongolism), occurring with an incidence of 1 in every 600 births throughout the world. Down syndrome is caused by the presence of one too many chromosomes. The normal complement of chromosomes is 46. Children with Down syndrome have 47 chromosomes.

The term mongolism was derived from facial features of children with Down syndrome, including upslanting eyelids and a depressed forehead. These children are always mentally retarded, but to different degrees. An adult with Down syndrome will usually function intellectually at a

2nd–6th grade level, with social functioning at a somewhat higher level. With recently developed therapy programs (infant stimulation and occupational and physical therapy), and better recognition of medical problems, such as hearing loss, the outcome will improve somewhat; but it is unlikely that a person with Down syndrome will be able to live completely independently. I tell parents of children with Down syndrome that the goal is for their child to be able to live in a sheltered home and to hold down an unskilled job.

Most special education and infant developmental programs will have several children with Down syndrome in attendance. In addition to mental retardation, half of all babies with Down syndrome have congenital heart disease, requiring heart surgery. About 10% of Down syndrome newborns have intestinal obstructions and require surgery. There is also an increased risk of congenital, or early occurring leukemia (a type of cancer of the blood) in children with Down syndrome.

Men with Down syndrome are almost always sterile. Therefore it is not necessary to be concerned about a male with Down syndrome fathering a child. I once received a call from a pediatrician who had scheduled a vasectomy for a sexually active young man with Down syndrome. Fortunately we were able to prevent this unnecessary surgery.

Women with Down syndrome are physically capable of having children. Since they have an abnormal number of chromosomes, such females are at high risk for having offspring with Down syndrome.

Down syndrome is usually caused by having an extra chromosome number 21. Instead of having two chromosome 21s, a patient with Down syndrome has three chromosome 21s. Therefore, the total number of chromosomes in a person with Down syndrome is usually 47. The usual karyotype of a girl with Down syndrome is 47,XX,+21, and a boy with Down syndrome is 47,XY,+21. Having three instead of two copies of an autosome is referred to as a trisomy. Therefore Down syndrome can also be called *trisomy 21.*

Trisomies are caused by a mistake that can occur during the production of the egg or sperm, or in the early cell divisions in the embryo. If the mistake occurs in the embryo, the resulting child may have two different types of cells in his body. The cells descended from cells resulting in defective division will have trisomy 21, but the progeny of cells from normal divisions will have a normal karyotype. Individuals who have more than one type of cell in their body are called *mosaics.* It is estimated that 2% of all people with Down syndrome are mosaic. The features of an individual with mosaic Down syndrome will depend on the percentage of normal cells and the percentage of trisomic cells in each organ. For example, if the brain has 80% normal cells, the individual would be expected to have less mental retardation that if he had 80% trisomic cells.

A child with mosaic Down syndrome may do much better intellectually than a child with non-mosaic trisomy 21. Unfortunately, there is no way to perform a karyotype on brain cells, so it is impossible to determine the percentage of trisomic cells in the brain of a person with mosaic Down syndrome.

The diagnosis of mosaic Down syndrome can be made if the usual karyotype of blood cells or skin cells reveals that some cells have 47 chromosomes and other cells are normal. However, even if these tests do not reveal any cells, the child may still have mosaic Down syndrome. *There is no medical way to prove that a child is* not *mosaic.* This is because we can only perform chromosome analysis on two types of cells, blood cells and skin cells. We can't perform a karyotype on brain cells or any other cell type in the body.

Many parents of children with Down syndrome cling to the hope that their child is mosaic, and therefore has a better prognosis than a child with non-mosaic Down syndrome. However, the distribution of normal and abnormal cells in the body of a child with mosaic Down syndrome is completely random.

I saw a six-month-old child with Down syndrome who was doing extremely well for a child affected with this disease. Eric was already sitting up unassisted and rolling over. I discussed the possibility of mosaicism with his parents and they were interested in pursuing the diagnosis. We performed a karyotype on Eric's blood cells and there were no normal cells. We then analyzed some skin cells, which revealed that 25% of his skin cells were normal. This proved that the child did, indeed, have mosaic Down syndrome. Eric is new five years old. He is mildly retarded with an IQ of 68. His parents are considering plastic surgery to eliminate the abnormal appearance of his eyes so he will not be stigmatized because he has Down syndrome.

You may hear about another type of Down syndrome called translocation Down syndrome. Translocation Down syndrome is caused by a different genetic mistake than the error in trisomy 21. Children with translocation Down syndrome are not clinically different from children with trisomy 21 Down syndrome. The diagnosis of translocation Down syndrome has important implications for the parents of the child and the siblings of the child with respect to their risks for having future children with Down syndrome, but does not alter the prognosis for the affected child.

Parents of children with triosomy 21 Down syndrome have a 1% risk of having another child with Down syndrome, whereas parents of children with translocation Down syndrome who are carriers of the translocations have a 10% risk of having another child with Down syndrome.

It is essential for children with Down syndrome to have close medical follow-up by either a geneticist or other specialist who is an expert in the care of handicapped children. This is because children with Down syndrome are likely to have other medical problems, such as hearing loss, dental problems, and orthopedic problems that require prompt recognition and intervention. For example, undetected and untreated hearing can lead to poor speech development.

A Word about Expectations for Children with Down Syndrome

If children with Down syndrome do not receive the special care they require, they usually function very poorly. Most people have encountered such an untreated individual in person or on television or depicted in literature. The stereotype most people have of a person with Down syndrome is someone with terrible posture (stooped shoulders), terrible dentition, indistinct speech, poor personal hygiene, shuffling gait, and salivation. This stereotype is unfortunate because it is not a true reflection of the capabilities of individuals with Down syndrome who receive the appropriate interventions. Because children with Down syndrome are easily recognized by their characteristic facial appearance, the incorrect stereotype of Down syndrome can result in a form of undeserved discrimination against individuals with Down syndrome.

I have noticed recent publicity campaigns that, I assume, are an attempt to combat this unfortunate image of children with Down syndrome. One poster shows an adolescent with Down syndrome sitting at a grand piano with the caption, "Don't be surprised"; another shows a young man with Down syndrome in a three piece suit, carrying a briefcase and walking next to an attractive young woman. I feel that, although these advertising campaigns are well intentioned, they are clearly misleading. I have no doubt that a child with Down syndrome can take piano lessons and learn to play simple pieces. The impression given by the poster picture is that a young man with Down syndrome has somehow become an accomplished pianist. This is not a reasonable expectation for a child with Down syndrome, and I would not only be surprised, I would be shocked to see a child with Down syndrome playing a Chopin nocturne.

The second picture is even more misleading. The poster implies that the young man has a white-collar job, walks to work carrying his briefcase, and has a close relationship with a pretty, nonretarded girlfriend. This is the cruellest image of them all. With maximum intellectual skills of an sixth-grader (12 years old) and social skills of an eighth grader (14 years old), this expectation is totally unrealistic. The optimum outcome for the overwhelming majority of children with Down syndrome is to hold an unskilled job. Their social and sex life will be with other retarded citizens.

Although these attempts to remove the public's inaccurate image of individuals with Down syndrome are well meaning, I feel that they are cruelly unrealistic and can lead to inappropriately high expectations for parents of children with Down syndrome.

Down syndrome is so common and its symptoms so well known that it is unlikely that a child with Down syndrome will go undiagnosed.

All the other disorders involving abnormal numbers of the autosomes (non-sex chromosomes) cause such severe mental dysfunction and physical abnormalities that it is almost inconceivable that such a child would escape detection.

However, there are over 100 syndromes involving the loss or gain of small amounts of autosomal chromosomal material that may cause subtle physical as well as mental abnormalities. These syndromes are named according to the type of chromosomal abnormality observed. *Deletions* involve the loss of genetic material; *duplications* involve additional genetic material. *Inversions, ring chromosomes,* and *unbalanced translocations* involve alterations in the structures of chromosomes. Any child with mental dysfunction who has *any* other physical abnormality or peculiar facial appearance should have a blood test called a karyotype performed to investigate the possibility of one of these chromosomal problems.

A mother brought in her six-year-old son who has a visual/perceptual learning disability. There are two older sisters in this family. The eldest daughter also has a learning disability. Her disability involves sequencing and letter recognition. As is discussed in Chapter 7, the same genetic disease can cause different patterns of mental handicap in different individuals. The occurrence of two siblings with mental dysfunction led me to do genetic tests. These revealed that both children were missing small amounts of one chromosome (called a deletion). This chromosomal abnormality was the cause of their problems.

Results of the parents' karyotype revealed that the father was a "carrier" for this chromosomal abnormality. This means that each of his children have about a 30% chance of inheriting the deletion and having mental dysfunction as the result. In addition, one-third of his children would be expected to be a carrier just like the father, and one-third of his children would be completely normal. Because of the possibility that their middle daughter was a carrier we tested her and she was, indeed, a carrier.

We explained to these parents that prenatal diagnosis could detect if an unborn child had inherited the deleted chromosome. We suggested that the parents consider this possibility for future pregnancies, and that the carrier daughter and the affected children consider the procedure when it was time for them to have children.

This information allowed the parents to have another child. Prior to the diagnosis, they had decided not to have more children because of the two children with disabilities. Because we were able to identify the cause of the learning disabilities in these children, the parents decided to have another child and utilize prenatal diagnosis. The prenatal diagnosis revealed a boy with normal chromosomes.

Sex Chromosome Abnormalities

In contrast to children with abnormal numbers of autosomes, children who have *abnormalities of the sex chro-*

mosomes may have subtle symptoms and are often not diagnosed until adolescence or adulthood. Sometimes the
diagnosis is not made during a person's lifetime, but is
discovered on autopsy. The sex chromosome abnormalities
that can cause mental dysfunction are Klinefelter's syndrome, XYY syndrome, XXX syndrome, and XXXX syndrome.

A different kind of sex chromosome abnormality
called the *Fragile X syndrome* is a combination of a sex
chromosome abnormality and an X-linked genetic disease.
Fragile X syndrome primarily affects boys, but girls can
also suffer from it.

Disorders involving abnormal numbers of sex chromosomes are the result of the same sort of mistake in
cell division that occurs in Down syndrome. These disorders do not have the global, devastating consequences of
the autosomal disorders, but nevertheless account for a
large amount of mental dysfunction and suffering.

Approximately 1 in 1000 males born will have two
X chromosomes and one Y chromosome instead of one
X and one Y chromosome. This disorder is called
Klinefelter's syndrome. Men with Klinefelter's syndrome are
generally tall with an average adult height of about 6 feet.
Other features of Klinefelter's syndrome are small testicles,
infertility, and incomplete development of secondary sex
characteristics (body hair, facial hair, penis size), and mental dysfunction. The average IQ of a man with Klinefelter's
syndrome is 90. Since the average IQ in the general population is 100, Klinefelter men have, on an average, significantly lower IQs than their normal counterparts.
However, since an IQ above 70 is considered in the nonretarded range, most individuals with Klinefelter's syn-

drome will not be classified as being mentally retarded. However, their genetic abnormality certainly causes a mental handicap. A child with Klinefelter's syndrome who otherwise would have an IQ of 120 may have an IQ of 110 because of his chromosomal abnormality, and a child who would otherwise be destined to have an IQ of 90 may have an IQ of 80 because of the extra X chromosome. In both cases the child would not be considered mentally retarded, but in both cases impairment of mental functioning has occurred.

In addition to the mild mental deficiency, there is a higher incidence of mental illness and criminal behavior in individuals with Klinefelter's syndrome. Institutions for the mentally retarded, institutions for the mentally ill, and prisons all have a five–tenfold higher incidence of Klinefelter syndrome than the general population.

It is important to put this observation in perspective. On the one hand, it is clear that having Klinefelter's syndrome places an individual at an increased risk of being in a mental institution or in prison; but on the other hand most men with Klinefelter's syndrome lead perfectly normal lives, with the exception of not being able to father children. As a matter of fact, the diagnosis of Klinefelter's syndrome is often made as the result of a couple's evaluation for infertility. The only observable dysfunction in these men is sterility.

The reason for this paradox is the following. The chances of any individual having significant mental illness is around 5 in 1000. A tenfold higher risk for men with Klinefelter's syndrome puts their risk at 5 per 100, or 5%. Therefore 95 out of 100 individuals with Klinefelter's syndrome will not have significant mental illness. Somehow, the extra X chromosome places Klinefelter males at *risk* for developing mental illness. We have yet to discover the mechanism of this phenomenon.

Rarely, a man is found to have the karyotype XXXY, or even XXXXY. All these men are considered to have Klinefelter's syndrome. The average intelligence of these men decreases with increasing numbers of X chromosomes. For example, the average IQ of a man with XXXY syndrome is 80, XXXXY is 70, etc.

Some men have the karyotype 47, XYY. There is no accepted name for this syndrome, although sometimes the inaccurate term "supermale" is used by the lay press to describe it. Prison populations have a higher incidence of men with this abnormality than is found in the general population. Like men with Klinefelter's syndrome, individuals with XYY tend to be tall and have mild mental dysfunction. The IQ of a child with XYY syndrome is, on average, 10–15 points lower than those of their unaffected siblings. Severe acne in childhood and adolescence is a frequent complication of XYY syndrome. The prevalence of XYY in institutionalized male juvenile delinquents is 1:35, 24 times the frequency of XYY in the general population.

Since the Y chromosome is only active in early prenatal life, and its only function, as noted, is to induce the formation of testicles, the concept that XYY individuals are somehow more virile or aggressive is absurd and inaccurate.

Because of the higher incidence of XYY and Klinefelter individuals in prison populations, it was once proposed that individuals with Klinefelter's syndrome and XYY were more prone to commit violent crime than the general population. During the time that this theory was popular, there was a rumor that Richard Specht, the convicted mass murderer of student nurses, had Klinefelter's syndrome or XYY, and that his defense attorney was going to argue that he was biologically driven to commit violent crime. He was tall and had severe acne as an adolescent, which would have been consistent with this notion, but I am not aware of any evidence to suggest that he actually had Klinefelter or XYY syndrome. A karyotype would have easily determined if this was the case.

There was also a rumor that executives of major corporations have a higher incidence of the XYY karyotype, but this has never been substantiated by any medical report.

Unlike men with Klinefelter's syndrome, XYY males have normal-sized testicles and are usually fertile. Because they have an abnormal number of sex chromosomes they are at high risk of fathering children with either Klinefelter's or XYY syndrome.

XXX Syndrome

Some females have an extra X chromosome (47,XXX). Since there is no Y chromosome present, these individuals are female. These girls usually appear normal in the first year of life, but often develop speech and language deficiencies, lack of coordination, poor academic performance, and immature behavior. Similar to Klinefelter males, XXX females tend to be taller than their chromosomally normal peers after puberty. Analogous to XXXY males, XXXX females have all the problems associated with XXX, but to a greater degree.

It is important to note that although individuals with the abnormal karyotypes 47,XXX, 47,XXY, and 47,XYY have average IQs lower than the average IQ of the general population, most of these individuals lead "normal lives." With the exception of the infertility in Klinefelter males (47,XXY), the majority of individuals with these disorders will be unaware of any ill effects from their chromosomal defect. The mental dysfunction may be subtle, and difficult to detect.

The same test, a karyotype, detects all the above mentioned chromosomal abnormalities. If you feel that your child may have one of these disorders, request that your doctor order a karyotype or see a geneticist.

Fragile X Syndrome (Martin-Bell Syndrome)

It has been recognized since the turn of the century that throughout the industrialized world, there are more retarded males than females. In the past, this phenomenon was attributed to differential expectations for male and female children, but the differences have continued despite the growing equality of the sexes.

Genetically, men differ from women in one important respect: women have two copies of all the genes on the X chromosome, whereas men have only one copy (because the Y chromosome only contains one gene). The X chromosome contains hundreds of genes that have no relation to gender, such as the gene whose deficiency causes the most common form of muscular dystrophy and the gene whose deficiency causes red-green color blindness. Therefore, if a woman has a defective gene on one of her X chromosomes, she has a normal gene on the other chromosome to compensate. However, if her son inherits her X chromosome containing the defective gene (a boy must inherit a Y chromosome from his father) he will not have a normal X chromosome to compensate for the defective gene and he will have a disease.

Using genetic reasoning, it was postulated that at least some of the excess of retarded boys was due to defective genes lying on the X chromosome. Geneticists sought out families with a medical history compatible with X-linked mental retardation with primarily males affected with inheritance through carrier females. Several families who exhibited X-linked mental retardation inheritance patterns were studied extensively. After years of investigation, it was discovered that in some of these families, when special karyotypes were performed on affected males, a fraction of their X chromosomes broke during the normal laboratory procedure. These X chromosomes that seemed more susceptible to breakage were called "fragile" X chromosomes.

Boys who have a fragile X chromosome are said to have *Fragile X syndrome.* The other name for this syndrome is *Martin-Bell syndrome.* Of boys with Fragile X syndrome, 80% have mental retardation or behavior problems. Approximately 20% of boys with Fragile X syndrome have behavior patterns including incessant motion, which leads to the incorrect diagnosis of infantile autism (see Chapter 2).

Since Fragile X syndrome has only been recognized in the United States for about 10 years, other symptoms of the disease are not well established. Large testicles and/or genitalia are present in many men with Fragile X syndrome after puberty, but many boys with this syndrome have normal testicular size and genitalia. I currently recommend that any boy with unexplained mental retardation and/or hyperkinetic or "autistic-like" behavior be tested for Fragile X syndrome.

Females have two X chromosomes. A woman who has one defective chromosome (i.e., a fragile X chromosome) and one normal chromosome is said to be a carrier female. Approximately 30% of carrier females who have one fragile X chromosome will be mentally retarded. The blood test for Fragile X syndrome is a special type of karyotype analysis. If an individual has Fragile X testing he will get a karyotype at the same time. However, individuals who have simply had a karyotype performed in the past will not have been tested for Fragile X syndrome.

Some children with the Fragile X syndrome are being treated with high doses of a vitamin known as folic acid. This treatment is experimental, and there is no good evidence to prove that it is beneficial for children with Fragile X syndrome. Chapter 12 has a discussion of mega-vitamin therapy for mentally handicapped children.

Treatment for Children with Chromosomal Diseases

Tremendous progress has been made in the nonspecific therapy of all children with mental retardation in terms of *occupational and physical therapy*, and *infant stimulation*. The use of these services, combined with better recognition and more aggressive treatment of medical problems (hearing loss, poor visual acuity, orthopedic, and dental problems) improves somewhat the prognosis for children with all forms of mental retardation, but will certainly not cure their diseases.

*No vitamin, allergic, or dietary therapy has proven ad-
vantageous to children with chromosomal disorders.*
Developing an understanding of the mechanism by
which abnormal amounts of genetic material lead to mental retardation is one of the most important scientific challenges in mental retardation research.

Polygenic (Multifactorial) Inheritance

The 1906 well-established genetic diseases listed in
Dr. McKusick's book are caused by genes and their action.
True genetic diseases are distinguished from diseases in
which genetic factors play a part in the causation of the
disorder, but are not totally responsible for the disease.
These diseases are called *genetically influenced diseases.*
Other names for this same phenomenon are *polygenic diseases* and *multifactorial diseases.*
Some birth defects are not caused by mutations in a
single gene, but clearly have some *genetic component* in
their causation. This conclusion derives from the fact that
certain birth defects are prone to occur repeatedly in families, but not with a high enough frequency to be considered purely genetic. These diseases include spina bifida,
most forms of congenital heart defects, schizophrenia, pyloric stenosis, and manic-depressive disorder.
In this type of birth defect there is an increased risk
of recurrence for a couple who have already had an affected
child. The recurrence risk for each of their future children
usually ranges between 3%–10%; the occurrence risk for
the general population is about 40 times less. In contrast,
the recurrence risk for an autosomal recessive disease is
25%. For dominant diseases where one parent is affected,

the recurrence risk is 50%. Therefore recurrence risks of 3%–10% cannot represent the action of a single gene. Perhaps a mutated gene provides a susceptibility to environmental damage or other problems. This is why I prefer the term *multifactorial* to *polygenic* for this type of inheritance.

I often read statements in newspapers or magazines that identify alcoholism, schizophrenia, and Alzheimer's disease as "genetic diseases." Then I will read that the "gene" for Alzheimer's disease or the "gene" for schizophrenia is being cloned by scientists. Such statements are inaccurate and definitely misleading. These conditions are not true genetic diseases, but are genetically *influenced* diseases. There is no single gene responsible for causing schizophrenia for the overwhelming majority of individuals afflicted with the disorder.

There are currently three scientific methods used to identify the influences of genetic factors in the cause of disease.

Finding a Genetic Marker

Sometimes a genetic test can identify genetic differences among individuals. If individuals of one group are more likely to have a disease than another group, this difference is called a genetic marker. In a true genetic disease, the genetic marker will actually allow prediction of individuals who will have the disease. In genetically influenced disorders, a genetic marker indicates genetic predisposition for this illness in the population.

Blood type is an example of a genetic marker. A blood test can determine whether your blood type is A, B, AB, or O. Your blood type is completely determined by your genes. Individuals with type O blood are slightly more likely to develop stomach ulcers than people with other blood types. The increased risk is quite small (1.3 to 1) but this is a well-established *genetic predisposition* to disease. However, *most* people with type O blood will not develop ulcers. If a blood-type O individual is not under stress, he will probably not develop an ulcer. However, if he is under stress, he is 30% more likely to develop an ulcer than a person with another blood type.

Klinefelter's syndrome is an example of a proven genetic *predisposition* to mental illness identified because of a genetic marker. In this case, the extra X chromosome is the genetic marker. Somehow, the extra X chromosome causing Klinefelter's syndrome puts an affected individual at an increased risk for developing mental illness, but it doesn't *cause* the mental illness. Most men with Klinefelter's syndrome do not have mental illness, but the extra X chromosome somehow makes them vulnerable to developing mental illness.

We do not yet know the mechanism by which the extra X chromosome in Klinefelter syndrome causes genetic susceptibility to mental illness. Men with Klinefelter's syndrome, in addition to having a higher risk of mental illness, also have lower IQs than the general population. This suggests that there may be some abnormality in brain structure in these men predisposing them to develop mental retardation and/or mental illness, but this remains an unproven theory. So, the question of how the extra X chromosome creates a genetic predisposition for the development of mental illness remains an unsolved mystery.

In the other examples we will discuss, genetic influences are *inferred* for one reason or another (usually because of recurrence of a disease within families or as the result of twin studies) but have not yet been proven.

Family Studies

Some diseases are more likely to recur within families than in the population at large. Results of these studies are often difficult to interpret because families share environmental and infectious exposures as well as genetic makeup. Statistical methods have been developed to analyze results from family studies to minimize the effect of nongenetic factors.

Spina bifida (meningomyelocele) is an example of this kind of disease. In spina bifida, the spinal canal fails to close during prenatal life. A genetic component to spina bifida is inferred from the observation that couples who have children with spina bifida are at an increased risk of having other children with spina bifida.

The risk of having a child with spina bifida in the general population in the United States is 1 in 200. If a couple has had a previous child with spina bifida their risk for each subsequent pregnancy is 10 times greater than the general population (1 in 20). If they have had two previously affected children their risk increases to 1 in 10 for each subsequent pregnancy. Spina bifida cannot be considered a genetic disease because the minimum recurrence risk in a genetic disease is 1 in 4 (for autosomal recessive genetic disease). Some genetic component appears to be operating to cause a predisposition to spina bifida. However, remembering our lesson from kuru we can't be absolutely sure that genes are involved at all.

Twin Studies

Identical twins are, by definition, genetically identical; each twin has exactly the same genetic composition. If one twin has a disease and the other does not, the disease cannot be 100% genetically caused. In genetic diseases, when one twin has a genetic disease his identical twin must also have that disease. Fraternal (nonidentical) twins do not have the same genetic composition, so they do not have to have the same genetic disease.

Caution must be used in interpreting twin data. If identical twins have the gene for retinoblastoma, it is possible that one could develop tumors and the other would not, even though we know that retinoblastoma is a genetic disease (see Chapter 3).

When environmental influences are believed to play a role in disease development, as in schizophrenia, it is extremely valuable to study identical twins who have been raised in different families. Such twin pairs are rare in the population, however, so that sufficient numbers for good statistical analysis are difficult to obtain.

One theory to explain genetic predisposition is the *multifactorial theory*. In this theory the diseases are called "multifactorial diseases" or "multifactorial diseases with a genetic component." This theory states simply that in genetically influenced diseases, the disease results from a combination of the genetic factors and nongenetic factors, such as the combination of genes and environment in retinoblastoma (see Chapter 3).

The *polygenic theory* postulates that genetically influenced diseases are the result of the combined action of several different genes. Since different genes are inherited independently, the polygenic disease theory explains the increased recurrence risks observed in families with genetically influenced diseases.

The terms multifactorial and polygenic are often used interchangeably, even though the two theories are not equivalent. It is important to remember that they are both *theories* developed to explain genetically influenced diseases. There is no conclusive evidence to prove either theory. It is probable that some genetically influenced diseases are multifactorial, some are polygenic, and others are a combination of both mechanisms.

The terms genetically influenced disease, polygenic disease, or multifactorial disease are used to describe diseases such as spina bifida, schizophrenia, alcoholism, pyloric stenosis, congenital heart disease, and manic depressive disorder that seem to have a genetic component.

Spina bifida is an easily definable physical deformity. One can determine whether or not an individual is affected by a physical examination and X rays. Disorders such as schizophrenia are much harder to diagnose, and often two physicians disagree about the diagnosis in a given individual. The subjectivity of psychiatric diagnosis creates tremendous problems in family and twin studies.

Another problem in determining the etiology (cause) of mental illnesses is that diseases such as schizophrenia may actually be combination of several different disorders, each caused by a different problem, but all leading to similar symptoms.

Some diseases are clearly genetic in some families but are not genetic in others. Schizophrenia, manic depressive disorder, and Alzheimer's disease are examples of such disorders.

Alzheimer's disease causes progressive mental deterioration and senility in adults. There are some families in the world known to have a genetic form of Alzheimer's disease. This is known because several family members in several generations of these families have early onset senility (40–55 years old). In some of these families, Alzheimer's disease has been proven to be linked to a single genetic marker on chromosome 21 (the chromosome involved in Down syndrome). This scientific discovery made the front page of newspapers around the country.

However, when other families with genetic Alzheimer's disease were studied, the disease was not linked to this marker. So, these families who have genetic Alzheimer's disease do not have the same defective gene and therefore have *different* genetic diseases with similar symptoms.

The overwhelming majority of cases of Alzheimer's disease are *not* caused by a single defective gene. Therefore when people talk about *the* gene for Alzheimer's disease, they really should be talking about *a* gene capable of causing symptoms resembling Alzheimer's disease in rare families. Although this gene is extremely interesting from a scientific standpoint in terms of understanding of the nature of Alzheimer's disease, there is not yet any clinical usefulness for this gene marker.

Following the newspaper stories describing the cloning of "the gene for Alzheimer's disease," I received several phone calls asking similar questions. "My father has Alzheimer's disease, can you do a test to determine if I'm going to get it?" Unfortunately I had to tell them that this discovery cannot help them.

Similarly, there are a small number of families in which schizophrenia is inherited in an autosomal dominant, genetic manner (inherited from parent to child to grandchild). As in Alzheimer's disease, these families differ in terms of the inheritance of genetic markers. The over-whelming majority of cases of schizophrenia are not ge-netic, but may be genetically influenced. Again, the newspaper stories reporting the cloning of "the gene for schizophrenia" gave false hope to family members and the millions who sufferer from schizophrenia.

Multiple Malformation Syndromes

Multiple malformation syndromes are disorders in which several birth defects occur together in the same combination in many individuals. For example, Down syn-drome is an example of a multiple malformation syndrome. In Down syndrome, individuals may have slanted eyes, small foreheads, small ears, mental retardation, heart de-fects, hearing problems, intestinal obstructions, eye abnor-malities, dental abnormalities, hand abnormalities, pelvis abnormalities, and poor muscle tone.

It is important to note that not all individuals with Down syndrome will have all of those birth defects. Listed in Table 7 are the percentages of patients with Down syn-drome who have the various problems.

It is not necessary for an individual to exhibit all of the features of Down syndrome in order to make the di-agnosis. Down syndrome is an example of a multiple mal-formation syndrome that is also a genetic disease. It is caused by the presence of an extra chromosome. The ge-netic test called a karyotype analyzes chromosomes and determines conclusively if an individual has Down syn-drome or other chromosome abnormality.

Although many multiple malformation syndromes are also genetic diseases, others are not genetically caused.

Table 7. Down Syndrome
Percentage of Patients with
Various Defects*

Mental retardation	99+%
Poor muscle tone	80%
Slanted eyes	80%
Small ears	60%
Hand abnormality	45%
Eye abnormalities	60%
Heart defects	40%
Intestinal obstruction	10%

*From Jones (1988).

There are no specific blood or X ray tests for most multiple malformation syndromes. Some multiple malformation syndromes, such as the fetal alcohol syndrome, are caused by prenatal exposure to harmful agents. This is discussed in my book *Have a Healthy Baby.*

Although the incidence of most genetic diseases and multiple malformation syndromes is usually rare, there are a tremendous number of different genetic diseases and multiple malformation syndromes. The British Columbia study of 1 million consecutive births determined the incidence of genetic disorders and nongenetic multiple malformation syndromes diagnosed before the age of 21 to be 7.9% (Baird *et al.*, 1988) (see Table 8).

It is important to note that this statistic is for all disorders and not just for those causing mental dysfunction.

Therefore, genetic diseases and multiple malformation syndromes have a great impact on society. In the United States there are approximately 3 million births each year. Therefore approximately 11,000 children will be born each

Table 8. Genetic Disorders and Nongenetic
Multiple Malformation Syndromes
Diagnosed Before Age 21*

Single gene:	Incidence/1,000 births
Autosomal recessive:	1.7
Autosomal dominant:	1.4
X-linked	0.5
Chromosomal disorders:	1.8
Polygenic/multifactorial	48.0
Multiple malformation syndromes	26.0
Total:	79.4 = 7.9%

*British Columbia study (Baird, 1988).

year with single gene genetic diseases and 5400 with chromosomal disorders. An additional 78,000 children will be born with polygenic disorders and 144,000 children will be born with nongenetic multiple malformation syndromes.

The next chapter describes symptoms frequently associated with genetic diseases. Specific genetic diseases and multiple malformation syndromes capable of causing or influencing mental dysfunction are discussed in subsequent chapters. As discussed in the Introduction, the recognition of these disorders is vital for the optimal medical, social, and educational care of a handicapped child.

Chapter 7

When to Suspect a Genetic Cause for Mental Dysfunction

There are many clues that suggest the presence of a genetic disease or a birth defect syndrome. Symptoms frequently associated with genetic disease and multiple malformation syndromes are listed below. Some of these symptoms indicate a particular type of disorder, whereas others are nonspecific. Any of these symptoms in a mentally handicapped child should be followed up by a complete genetic evaluation. Ask your doctor for a referral to a clinical geneticist, or you can contact the American Society of Human Genetics in Rockville, Maryland for a listing of board-certified geneticists in your area and their qualifications. See Thompson and Thompson (1986), Strom (1988), Emery and Rimoin (1982), and Jones (1988) for further details.

More Than One Family Member Affected

One of the first things I do as a geneticist when I see a new patient is find out about every individual in the patient's extended family. Each of the three major classes of genetic diseases (*dominant*, *recessive*, and *X-linked*; see Chapter 6) has its own special pattern of inheritance. Since some genetic diseases can be quite variable in their symptoms, different individuals in the same family who are affected with the same genetic disease may be affected to varying degrees. For example, it is possible for one sibling with Fragile X syndrome to have profound mental retardation, while another sibling with the same syndrome may not be retarded but may have a behavioral problem.

The following is a discussion of the most common relationships in genetic diseases.

More Than One Sibling Affected

If two or more siblings have similar problems, there is a good chance that the problems are due to a genetic disease or multiple malformation syndrome. Although it is possible that the children were affected by the same environmental agent, such as lead poisoning or child abuse, a genetic evaluation is in order. This evaluation may reveal that the siblings suffer from a genetic disease, or it may reveal another medical cause for their problems.

I saw two sisters in clinic. The older girl, Pamela, was a mentally retarded six-year-old with an IQ of 60.

The younger sister, Roberta, was three years old and had not yet begun to talk. There was also an eight-year-old brother with no problems and an 18-month-old sister who was already talking. Both parents were of Swedish ancestry. Since birth, both Pamela and Roberta suffered from nearly continuous problems with skin rashes and eczema. Pamela was extremely short with respect to her classmates. I was able to make the diagnosis of a genetic disease called *Sjögren-Larsson syndrome* in these sisters. This is a recessive genetic disease that occurs primarily in people of Swedish ancestry. This disease causes mental retardation, skin problems, and short stature (height). Because this is an *autosomal recessive* genetic disease, each child of this couple has a one-in-four risk for Sjögren-Larsson syndrome.

Sometimes no genetic factors are involved, but siblings can have similar problems because they live in the same house and are exposed to the same environmental hazards.

I evaluated two siblings for attention deficit disorder. Linda was in the fourth grade and had previously been doing well in school. Her school performance began deteriorating about six months prior to her evaluation. Her seven-year-old brother, Philip, was in the first grade, had trouble sitting still in class and was performing poorly. Psychological testing revealed that both children had performance and verbal IQ's in the above-average range, with performance IQ lower than the verbal IQ (see Chapter 1).

In interviewing the parents I learned that they had begun home remodeling during the summer before school started. They often worked at night, scraping off old paint during the evenings and weekends when the children were in the house. I suspected lead poisoning, and blood tests confirmed that both children were suffering from mild cases of lead poisoning. After six weeks of treatment, their mental function began to improve and after six months, Linda was able to progress normally in school. Philip continues to have a residual learning disability, probably as the result of permanent brain damage caused by lead poisoning.

Toxic exposures can also occur while the fetus is still in the womb. I was asked to evaluate two siblings for developmental delay and mental retardation. After examining them I was convinced that they both suffered from *fetal alcohol syndrome*. In fetal alcohol syndrome, prenatal damage occurs due to alcohol ingestion by the mother during pregnancy. I asked this mother if she had done much drinking during her pregnancies. Her answers made it clear that she was an alcoholic and had consumed large amounts of alcohol during both pregnancies. After explaining that her drinking had damaged her children, we were able to convince her to enter a detoxification program. Unfortunately nothing can reverse the brain damage in her two children.

Often two children with the same exposures or the same genetic disease exhibit different symptoms. For example, one sibling may be developmentally delayed while another may be learning disabled. When two or more siblings suffer from mental dysfunction, regardless of the exact nature of the mental dysfunction, they should be medically and genetically evaluated. The forms of mental dysfunction may be developmental delay, mental retardation, mental illness, emotional disorder, learning disability, attention deficit disorder, or neurological disability.

*Son Affected; also Mother's Brother, Father,
Grandfather, or Sister's Son*

This is the classic inheritance pattern of an *X-linked* genetic disease.

I saw 12-year-old Alan in genetics clinic. He was identified as mentally retarded with emotional problems in kindergarten. He has two older sisters with normal intelligence. Alan's mother has a mentally retarded brother and two of her sisters have five sons who are mentally retarded. Genetic testing confirmed a diagnosis of Fragile X syndrome (see Chapter 6). When Alan's uncle and all the affected cousins were tested, all had the Fragile X syndrome. Since Fragile X syndrome is an X-linked genetic disease, each son of carrier mothers will have a 50% chance of having Fragile X syndrome.

Alan's mother's other sisters, who had not yet had children, were tested, and one of them is a carrier for Fragile X syndrome. Her future sons also have a 50% risk of having the disease.

There is currently no effective medical treatment for Fragile X syndrome. If this family had known about their genetic problem, they could have utilized prenatal diagnosis or made different decisions regarding family planning.

Any time a boy is affected with mental dysfunction and he has a brother, maternal uncle, paternal grandfather, or male cousin (his mother's sister's son) also affected with any kind of mental dysfunction, a genetic and medical evaluation is needed. In addition, because of the frequency of Fragile X syndrome (1 in 1000 boys), any boy with unexplained mental dysfunction (no apparent cause of the dysfunction, see Chapter 5) should be tested for Fragile

X syndrome, especially if any symptoms of hyperactivity or autistic-like symptoms are present.

One Parent and One or More Children Affected

This is the characteristic inheritance pattern of *autosomal dominant* genetic diseases. It is quite common for one of the parents of a child with a learning disability to have had school problems. If you are a teacher, you will usually need to ask very specific questions. This information is rarely offered, because people often feel embarrassed about a learning handicap, even though they have overcome the handicap and are successful. It is possible for a person with a significant learning disability to succeed in business despite his or her handicap.

The most common familial form of primary learning disability is inherited from one parent to a child. In these families the learning disability is inherited in a genetically dominant manner. In a dominant genetic disease, each child of an affected parent has a 50-50 chance of inheriting the defective gene and being affected themselves.

When I interview parents I always ask, "Did either of you have any problems in school?" and "How far did you get in school?"

Never assume that because an individual is successful or articulate that he or she does not have a learning disability. This lesson was brought home to me during one interview.

Both parents brought six-year-old Todd to see me because of problems with attention span and behavior that had suddenly appeared in the first grade.

Todd's mother was elegantly dressed and wore several thousand dollars worth of jewelry. His father was a vice president of a major multinational electronics corporation. Taking my own advice, I asked my questions. I was stunned by the father's response.

"Funny you should ask," he said. "I was never able to learn how to read in elementary school and I dropped out after the fourth grade. When I was 13, I lied about my age and got a job as an errand boy for the sales department in my company. The guys helped me learn how to fill in the sales reports, and they read the sales literature to me and I memorized it. I eventually became all-time sales leader for the Midwest district. I was eventually able to learn to read the newspaper, but I still had to have people read me complicated things like sales brochures and employee benefit pamphlets.

"I could sell anyone anything and was very popular among my colleagues. One day, after a merger, an executive asked me if I would like a promotion to become a sales manager. He said I would have my own secretary. I was nervous, but I said OK. Everyone in the sales department already knew about my reading problems, and they were extremely supportive. My secretary would spend hours reading to me and eventually we designed a system where she filled in the numbers in a standardized form, so I could "read" the monthly salesmen's reports.

"Writing was now no problem because I could dictate everything. Everything went smoothly and I have done quite well."

Todd's father is obviously very smart and he was able to overcome his disability. Todd inherited the same learning disability, dyslexia (reading disability) from his father. This sort of dominantly inherited learning disability is the most common form of inherited learning disability.

Although there is no specific medical treatment for the dominantly inherited genetic learning disability that Todd and his father have, it is important to make the diagnosis so that parents can be counseled as to the recurrence risk for future children. The affected child will also have a 50-50 chance of passing on the defective gene to each of his or her future children.

Todd's educational testing revealed a very high IQ and a profound learning disability in letter recognition and reversal. His tutor and I designed a program of tapes and supportive remediation so that Todd, unlike his father, would not have to drop out of elementary school. Todd's parents were very grateful, and relieved. Since the father had succeeded, they were confident that Todd would succeed as well.

There are other autosomal dominant genetic diseases that can cause mental dysfunction.

I evaluated Hal, a nine-year-old child with a learning disability, in clinic. His father was a salesman for a local company. When I asked Hal's father my usual questions, he told me that he had dropped out of high school in the tenth grade because he had so much trouble reading. Eventually, he earned his high school equivalency diploma and worked his way up in his company. Both Hal and his father were extremely tall, and nearsighted. Hal's father needed a hearing aid. After examining both of them, I determined that they both suffered from a disease known as Stickler's disease which causes joint problems, nearsightedness, progressive hearing loss, and mental dysfunction. Since this is a dominant genetic disease, each of Hal's father's children will have a 50-50 chance of having Stickler's disease.

Because of the diagnosis of Stickler's disease, Hal's hearing was checked, and he also requires a hearing aid which has helped him function better in class. Hal's parents were relieved to know the reason for their son's problems.

All children with mental dysfunction who have a parent affected with mental dysfunction should have a genetic and medical evaluation.

Previous Stillbirths, Miscarriages, or Unexplained Deaths of Children of Either Parent

The same genetic disease can affect children differently. The disease may cause a miscarriage, stillbirth, or death in infancy in one child and only intermittent illness and mild mental dysfunction in a sibling.

If a sibling has died of an unexplained illness, and the child in question has mental handicaps, a genetic evaluation is necessary. In such a case, establishing a diagnosis may allow medical intervention that can prevent life-threatening future complications.

I was called to see six-year-old Michael, who was in a coma. The boy was in a special education class because of a learning disability. Throughout his life, Michael had frequent episodes of vomiting during which he would get very sleepy. He had had a brother who began vomiting on his third day of life and then lapsed into a coma and died. Genetic testing of Michael revealed that he had an *X-linked* genetic disease called ornithine transcarbamylase deficiency. Children with this disease are not able to digest protein properly. The intermittent problems with vomiting and sleepiness were due to the buildup of toxins in his body because of his disease. These episodes caused permanent brain damage resulting in Michael's learning disability.

After the toxins were removed from his bloodstream he woke up and was placed on a special low-protein diet and medication was prescribed to help remove the poisons from his body. Although he hasn't had any more attacks of vomiting or coma, Michael's mental disability remains. Much of his brain damage might have been prevented if the diagnosis had been made sooner.

His parents were informed of the recurrence risk of X-linked diseases: each son has a 50% risk of having the disease, and a 50% chance of being normal, and each daughter has a 50% chance of being a carrier for the disease.

The brother who died in infancy in this family almost certainly also had ornithine transcarbamylase deficiency, but was much more severely affected. In this disease, carrier females can also be affected. Michael's sister was tested and was found not to be a carrier of ornithine transcarbamylase deficiency.

There are other symptoms in addition to family recurrences that point to a medical cause for mental disability.

Polyhydramnios (Too Much Amniotic Fluid)

In the womb, the fetus is surrounded by a liquid called amniotic fluid. Amniotic fluid is continually produced by the baby's kidneys. Since there is continuous production of fluid there must also be a way to get rid of the fluid. This is done by the baby swallowing the amniotic fluid. Once swallowed, the fluid is absorbed from the baby's stomach and intestines into the baby's bloodstream. From there, the fluid is either taken away by the mother's blood through the placenta or is used by the baby's kidneys to make urine and subsequently make more amniotic fluid. Abnormalities of brain function in the baby can cause a reduction in the amount and rate of swallowing. This can lead to buildup of too much amniotic fluid (polyhydramnios).

Polyhydramnios can be diagnosed during pregnancy if the size of the womb increases faster than usual, or it can be detected during an ultrasound examination. Intestinal obstructions can also lead to polyhydramnios.

A history of polyhydramnios in a child with mental handicap indicates that the brain dysfunction began prenatally. A medical and genetic evaluation is needed because the history of polyhydramnios suggests a physical cause for the mental disability. Polyhydramnios does not *cause* brain injury; prenatal brain abnormalities cause polyhydramnios. There is no treatment for polyhydramnios.

I evaluated Angela, an eight-year-old girl with mild mental retardation and social problems. Her mother told me that during her pregnancy she grew so big that an ultrasound was performed. It showed polyhydramnios. When Angela was evaluated at 18 months of age for developmental delay, the mother was told that Angela's problems were due to poor parenting. This unfortunate mother had carried an unnecessary burden of guilt for many years. I was able to tell her that Angela's mental dysfunction began in the womb and therefore her daughter's dysfunction could not have been caused by bad parenting.

Genetic testing revealed that Angela actually had a small chromosomal deletion which was the cause of the polyhydramnios and her subsequent mental handicap.

Loss of Developmental Milestones

Children with mental retardation develop more slowly than "normal" children. Like "normal" children they attain developmental milestones such as rolling over, sitting up, crawling, and walking in the expected order, but at later times than a "normal" child.

Once retarded children attain a skill, they continue to have that skill. Children who begin to lose the ability to do physical and/or mental tasks that they could previously perform may suffer from a genetic disease. More than 20 different genetic diseases cause progressive mental and/or neurological deterioration. A child who begins to lose developmental milestones needs prompt evaluations by a neurologist and a geneticist.

True loss of developmental milestones should not be confused with regression. Sometimes children regress following an emotional or physical trauma, but these regressions usually involve social, toilet training, and verbal skills. Regression is usually *transient* and children usually regain the skill within a short time. Psychotherapy can be very helpful in this situation. As noted in Chapter 2, loss of developmental milestones is not transient; deterioration is progressive.

A mother brought her 16-year-old son Larry to see me because of progressive mental deterioration. In the seventh grade he had been at the top of his class and was getting straight A's. In the eighth grade he starting getting

B's. In the ninth grade he got C's and in the tenth grade he was failing all his subjects. Even more striking were the yearly photographs taken on his birthdays. At 13 Larry had been a bright-eyed, alert child. Each year he deteriorated, so that by his 15th birthday the photograph clearly showed a retarded teenager. During this period Larry lost the ability to ride a bicycle and became progressively more clumsy. Genetic testing revealed that Larry has a genetic disease called metachromatic leukodystrophy, a degenerative neurological disease. Fortunately for this family, none of the other 3 children suffered from this disease, although it is an *autosomal recessive genetic disease* (each had a one in four risk of having the disease).

This family decided to try a bone marrow transplant for their son in an attempt to arrest the progression of this otherwise degenerative and fatal disease.

If untreated, Larry would probably die within the next 10 years. It is not yet known whether the transplant will arrest the degenerative process, but a transplant will probably not reverse the damage that has already occurred. If the diagnosis had been made when Larry was younger, the transplant might have been performed sooner and perhaps he would have done better.

Other Indications

Unusual Odor

Inborn errors of metabolism or *inherited metabolic diseases* can involve defects in the body's ability to prevent the buildup of various toxic substances (see Chapters 9 and 10).

In many of these diseases, toxic compounds build up in the body and give the body and/or urine an unusual odor. For example, in the disease isovaleric acidemia, a substance called isovaleric acid builds up in the body. Children with isovaleric acidemia excrete large amounts of isovaleric acid into their urine, giving their urine the distinctive smell of sweaty socks. There is even a disease named maple syrup urine disease because the urine of children with the disease smells like maple syrup; and I can assure you that it really does!

Phenylketonuria (PKU) is an inborn error of metabolism that, if untreated, leads to irreversible, profound mental retardation. Children with PKU are unable to digest proteins properly. A toxic substance builds up in their bodies and injures their growing brains.

The recognition of the cause of mental retardation in PKU and its treatment represent the first successful prevention of mental retardation in the history of medicine.

The discovery was made in the 1950s by a chemist who recognized the smell of the abnormal chemical in the diapers of institutionalized retarded children. The odor was so strong and distinctive that the nurses of the institution had placed all the infants with PKU in a single nursery even though they had no idea that the children all had the same genetic disease! The doctor/chemist also noticed that all the children had fair complexions and blue eyes (two other features of PKU). He went on to analyze their urine and thereby made one of the most important discoveries in the history of genetics. Children with PKU can be treated with a low-protein diet that completely prevents mental retardation (see Chapter 12).

It is not necessarily a strong smell, but an unusual smell that is the clue in organic acidemias. Urine can smell strong simply because it is concentrated, but it will still smell like normal urine. The following is a list of unusual urine odors known to be associated with genetic diseases:

Musty
Maple syrup or burnt sugar
Dried malt or hops
Boiled cabbage or rancid butter
Cheesy
Sweaty feet or socks
Cat urine

If you notice one of these unusual odors to the urine or sweat of a child with mental dysfunction, take the child immediately to a geneticist for a biochemical evaluation.

Unusual Color to the Urine

There is a fascinating subset of metabolic genetic diseases called the *porphyrias* that can cause intermittent abdominal pain and symptoms such as paranoia, insomnia, seizures, and epilepsy. Patients with porphyrias have large amounts of abnormal chemicals in their urine that can turn red or reddish-brown after exposure to light, heat, or acids. If you see a red color in a used diaper or in an unflushed toilet, this may be caused by these compounds. The diagnosis of a porphyria is extremely important because the symptoms may be preventable. Many people may be classified as being hysterical or mentally ill when they actually have a genetic inherited metabolic disease.

Abnormal Skin Blistering or Rashes

The porphyrias (see above section and Chapter 8) can also lead to extreme sensitivity of the skin to sunlight. If an individual requires copious amounts of sun block to avoid blistering in the sun, he or she should be evaluated for porphyria (special urine and blood tests). Other genetic diseases such as Sjögren-Larsson disease involve severe eczema in association with mental retardation. Intense freckling can also be associated with mental retardation in a disorder known as DiSanctis Cocchione syndrome.

Another inborn error of metabolism called multiple carboxylase deficiency can result in recurrent yeast infections of the skin and developmental delay. The symptoms resemble recurring eczema or psoriasis.

Children with recurrent skin rashes, eczema, unusual freckling, or other skin abnormalities should be evaluated by a geneticist.

Unusual Consistency or Color of Hair

Some inborn errors of metabolism result in brittle or dry hair. Extremely fair hair may indicate a biochemical problem with the production of pigment. One of these diseases, phenylketonuria (PKU) can result in profound mental retardation if not treated in infancy (see above).

There is also a genetic disease that results in extremely fragile and curly hair called *Menke's syndrome*. This disease causes severe developmental delay and usually results in death prior to age six years.

Hair Loss (Alopecia)

Some inherited metabolic diseases cause hair to fall out. Usually parents notice that tufts of hair fall out while combing their child's hair. Bald patches may develop on the scalp.

If children with mental dysfunction have any problems with excessive hair loss or an unusual consistency or brittleness to their hair, a genetic evaluation is needed.

Abnormal Eye Movements

There are many different kinds of abnormal eye movements. Crossed eyes, wandering eyes, and nystagmus are the most common. In nystagmus, the eyes jerk rapidly and repeatedly in one direction. Nystagmus is normal when looking at a moving train, but is usually abnormal under circumstances when the child is not looking at a moving object. There are many possible medical causes of abnormal eye movements, including blindness, nearsightedness, farsightedness, amblyopia (lazy eyes), and muscle weakness. Any abnormal eye movements in an infant or child should be evaluated by an ophthalmologist immediately. Failure to obtain the appropriate diagnosis can result in permanent vision impairment.

Recurrent Episodes of Vomiting without Diarrhea

Many of the inherited metabolic diseases (see Chapter 10) produce symptoms intermittently. Toxins build up in the body because of the body's inability to digest protein properly, and this buildup causes nausea and vomiting. The vomiting in children with inborn errors of metabolism is episodic. The episodes can be triggered by viral infections such as colds or flu accompanied by fever. Children with an inborn error of metabolism often have vomiting and fever, the identical symptoms of children with gastroenteritis.

Usually the treatment for vomiting episodes is to place the child on a clear liquid diet. Clear liquids have no protein, and since these metabolic diseases involve protein intolerance, the clear liquid diet leads to an improvement of the symptoms. Since vomiting in a child with a metabolic disease is not caused by an infection, there will usually be no diarrhea during these episodes. This is in contrast to the usual episodes of gastroenteritis (stomach flu) in children; gastroenteritis causes diarrhea with or without vomiting as the primary symptoms.

Children with inborn errors of metabolism can have recurrent episodes of vomiting as often as once a month or as infrequently as once or twice a year. Sometimes during these episodes the child becomes sleepy or "lethargic" and can progress to coma.

I evaluated Marie, a three-year-old child with developmental delay. Her parents told me that approximately once a month Marie would get the "stomach flu" and begin vomiting. These episodes were treated with a clear liquid diet and resolved within two to three days. Various doctors had attributed these episodes to emotional stress, repeated infections, or gastrointestinal abnormalities. Genetic testing revealed that Marie suffered from an inherited metabolic disease known as *multiple carboxylase deficiency* which can be treated with a vitamin known as biotin. Biotin treatment not only eliminated the vomiting episodes, but improved her developmental and neurological function.

Any child with mental dysfunction who has recurrent episodes of "stomach flu" with vomiting as a prominent feature should be referred to a geneticist for evaluation. (See Chapter 10 for further discussion of multiple carboxylase deficiency.)

Recurrent Episodes of Sleepiness, Lethargy, or Coma

Children with inborn errors of metabolism may have repeated episodes of sleepiness, or be extremely difficult to wake up. These are not children who simply have difficulty getting up in the morning. These symptoms refer to children who cannot be aroused at all or who, after arousal, immediately return to sleep despite vigorous stimulation. (See discussion of isovaleric acidemia and multiple carboxylase deficiency, Chapters 6 and 10.)

Unusual Food Preferences or Avoidance

Some inborn errors of metabolism interfere with normal digestion of certain food products. Children with some of these diseases may avoid certain foods because when they eat them they experience unpleasant side effects such as nausea.

There is a famous picture of a six-year-old boy who was handed an apple to eat. He ate only the skin and left the entire pulp untouched. He did not know it at the time, but he had an autosomal recessive genetic disease called *hereditary fructose intolerance.* This disease causes an inability to digest fructose (the sugar found in fruit pulp) and if untreated can lead to brain damage and seizures. An interesting fact about hereditary fructose intolerance is that no child with this disease has ever had a single dental cavity because of their nearly total avoidance of sugar.

Protein avoidance is another clue that a child may have an inborn error of metabolism. I remember a six-year-old girl with a disease called *propionic acidemia,* a disorder of faulty protein digestion. Her mother told me that it took three people to get her to drink her milk, two to hold her down and one to hold her nose and pour the milk down. This girl also had recurrent episodes of vomiting and suffered from a learning disability, probably as the result of brain damage occurring during these episodes.

Therefore, protein avoidance (milk, meat) or sugar avoidance may be a clue that a child suffers from an inborn error of metabolism.

Facial or Other Physical Appearance Unlike Parents or Siblings

Children with the same genetic disease or birth defect syndrome resemble each other much more than they resemble their parents, siblings, or other relatives. Sometimes the child with the handicap looks totally different from any of the other family members. This phenomenon can be so striking that I can recognize a child with a genetic disease as soon as the family walks into my office. If a nonadopted child looks physically much different from any of his or her relatives, the child may have a genetic disease or multiple malformation syndrome.

I had just given a lecture to a parents' group for learning-disabled children. In the lobby outside the auditorium, I noticed a woman standing with four children. Three of the children resembled the mother, with delicate features and fair complexions. The fourth child, however, had extremely coarse features, and thick-looking skin. Fortunately this woman approached me to ask me a question. During our conversation I was able to determine that all four children were hers and that they had the same father. The fourth child had mild mental retardation. I recommended a genetic evaluation for this child, and subsequent genetic testing revealed that the child suffered from a genetic disease called *Hunter's disease*. The original name for Hunter's disease was *gargoylism*, because individuals with this disorder develop facial features reminiscent of gargoyles.

Children with Hunter's disease suffer from progressive brain damage and can also have instability in their spinal columns.

Although there is no treatment for Hunter's disease to prevent the progressive brain damage, steps can be taken to prevent any paralysis due to dislocations of the spine. For this family, establishing the diagnosis of Hunter's syndrome was important for several reasons. We were able to explain the basis of the child's problems and tell the his parents what to expect in his future and how to prevent major secondary complications such as paralysis.

This couple wanted more children. Since Hunter's disease is an X-linked genetic disease, each son is at 50% risk of having the disease. This couple chose to use prenatal diagnosis for their next pregnancy; when the test revealed a male fetus with Hunter's disease, they terminated this pregnancy. A prenatal diagnosis for the next pregnancy revealed an unaffected boy, who was born healthy and is doing well. Therefore, establishing the diagnosis of Hunter's disease in this child had beneficial effects for this family.

Consanguinity

Consanguinity is the medical term used when two blood relations have children together. Consanguinity creates a high risk of producing a child with a genetic disease. Consanguinity frequently occurs in certain closed societies such as the Amish and Appalachians who intermarry according to custom. Consanguinity may be the result of incest.

If a mental disability is present in a child of a consanguineous couple, a genetic evaluation is necessary.

Short Stature (Height)

There are many genetic diseases that cause mental dysfunction and also cause children to grow poorly. If a child is shorter than other children his age *and* has mental handicaps, a genetic evaluation is necessary. However, most dwarfing conditions do not cause mental dysfunction.

Accelerated Growth

One particular multiple malformation syndrome, called cerebral gigantism (Soto's syndrome), causes accelerated growth and maturation and mental retardation and/or learning disability. Children who are very large for their age may be suffering from this disease and need a genetic evaluation.

"Organic" Behavioral or Learning Problems

Many experienced health care workers and educators recognize some children who do not fit the usual mold. They often refer to these children as being "organic." This term comes from the medical term "organic brain syndrome," which refers to psychiatric symptoms of physical origin.

An "organic" child may very well have a genetic disease and can benefit from a genetic evaluation.

Presence of Other Birth Defects

Children with mental handicaps who also have other birth defects may have a birth defect syndrome and will benefit from a genetic evaluation. Although it would be impossible to list all of the possible birth defects that may occur with mental disability in a multiple malformation syndrome, some of the most common are listed (Jones, 1988):

Cleft lip and/or palate
Webbed or extra fingers or toes
Spine abnormalities (curvature or abnormal bone
    structure)
Undescended testicles

Abnormally shaped or positioned ears
Loose joints
Abnormal body proportions
Dislocated lenses or severe near-sightedness
Heart problems (holes in the heart, abnormal
    heart structure)
Short jaw
Slanted eyes (with non-Asian parents)
Cataracts
Absence of or poorly developed teeth
Tall stature
Short stature
Kidney problems
Abnormally shaped head
Abnormal hair loss (alopecia)

Chapter 8

Diseases Causing Specific
Behavioral Patterns

In Chapter 3 we discussed the concepts of nature and nurture in the context of the causes of mental disability. Certain very rare genetic diseases cause specific stereotypic behaviors; these genetic diseases actually cause the same abnormal behavioral pattern in almost all children affected with the disease. These rare diseases produce behaviors that are totally, or nearly totally, nature-caused. Although scientists have been studying these diseases carefully for clues to the biological cause of behavior, we still do not understand why these diseases cause these specific behaviors. For additional information regarding these disorders see Thompson and Thompson (1986), Scriver et al. (1989), and Jones (1988).

This chapter identifies rare *genetic diseases, multiple malformation syndromes, chromosomal defects,* and *toxins* that cause specific abnormal behaviors. *Lesch-Nyhan syndrome* is an example of a genetic disease in which "nature" contributes nearly 100% to behavioral abnormalities. *Congenital indifference to pain, Williams syndrome, Cornelia de Lange syndrome, porphyria, Wilson's Disease,* and *Tourette's syndrome* are genetic diseases in which "nature" contributes to mental dysfunction. Multiple malformation syndromes that have identifiable, "nature-caused" mental and physical abnormalities include Prader-Willi syndrome, Laurence-Moon-Biedle syndrome, Bardet-Biedl syndrome, Börjeson-Forssman-Lehmann syndrome, Carpenter's syndrome, Cohen syndrome, and Killian-Teschler-Nicola syndrome. Chromosomal diseases with a "nature-caused" component of mental dysfunction include Klinefelter's syndrome, XYY syndrome, and XXX syndrome; these were mentioned in the section on genetically influenced disorders in Chapter 6.

Lesch-Nyhan Syndrome: Self-Mutilation

The classic disease in which genetic defects cause a specific abnormal behavior pattern is an X-linked genetic disease called Lesch-Nyhan syndrome. This disease is caused by a deficiency of a single protein in the body, an enzyme called hypoxanthine-guanine-phosphoribosyl-transferase, or HGPRT for short. Enzymes are proteins in the body that are responsible for performing one of the thousands of specific chemical reactions necessary to sustain normal life. In a genetic disease such as Lesch-Nyhan syndrome, an inherited metabolic disease, one of the thousands of enzymes in the body is defective and cannot do its job, so the body cannot perform one specific chemical reaction. One way to understand the consequences of such a deficiency is to think of a roadblock. A roadblock on a busy highway will create a tremendous traffic jam. Depending on the location of the barrier, there may be exits or side streets that can provide alternative routes and alleviate some of the backup. However, if the roadblock is on a bridge, there will be no way to bypass the barrier and reach the destination.

Patients with Lesch-Nyhan syndrome appear completely normal at birth. In infancy, they are usually slow to develop physical skills and they become spastic (stiff muscles). Later on, they all become plagued by compulsions to self-mutilate and to injure others. Their arms and legs must be restrained at all times or else the affected boys (since this disease is X-linked, only boys are affected) chew off their lips, the ends of their fingers and toes, and hit themselves and others to the point of serious injury. As soon as the diagnosis of Lesch-Nyhan syndrome is made, the central incisor teeth must be pulled to prevent the boys from completely chewing off their lips and biting off the ends of their tongues. These children also have compulsions to strike out and hurt others, even those they love. They will bite, punch, slap, and spit at loved family members as well as medical and nursing staff. In adolescence they are often verbally abusive, often shocking people with prodigious displays of profanity and insults.

Although many textbooks report that boys with Lesch-Nyhan syndrome are severely retarded, my personal experience is that they are usually of at least average intelligence. However, because of their physical limitations and compulsive, uncontrollable (except for the use of restraints) abusive behavior, they are extraordinarily difficult to educate.

When boys with Lesch-Nyhan syndrome are not in the grips of a compulsion, they can be quite pleasant to be with. It is extremely poignant to discuss their compulsions with them.

One of my favorite patients with Lesch-Nyhan syndrome is a young man I will call Calvin. Calvin and I met while I was doing my pediatric internship and we became good friends. Once when I was examining him in clinic and he was momentarily unrestrained (so that I could examine his abdomen) he suddenly blurted out the words "Hold me." Before I could figure out what he meant he had delivered a blow to my face that broke my glasses. Then he proceeded to hit himself repeatedly in the groin until I could, with help, restrain him. I asked Calvin if he was mad at me, or if he would like another doctor to take care of him. He told me that he still liked me a lot and he wasn't mad at me—he just gets an urge he can't resist.

He then confided to me that this episode was different from his usual encounters with his speech therapist (who had complained to me that Calvin spit at her). He said he didn't like his therapist, so he continually spat at her. He was clever enough to realize that no one would get mad at him for spitting because they would blame it on his disease. I asked Calvin if he could feel it when he bit or hit himself; did he feel pain or pleasure? He answered that it hurt him very much, but he just couldn't stop doing it.

I do not think Calvin is mentally retarded. Obviously, it is difficult to educate a child who needs continual restraint to prevent him from hurting himself and others, who spits, and is verbally abusive. Calvin attends school, knows how to read, and he is an avid San Diego Padres baseball fan. He can't learn to write because he is extremely spastic and is in restraints all the time to prevent him from hurting himself.

Another boy with Lesch-Nyhan syndrome was undiagnosed until he was eight years old. When I first saw him and made the diagnosis of Lesch-Nyhan syndrome he was in a behavior modification program and was continually receiving "negative reinforcement" (punishments) for his "aggressive" and "self-destructive" behaviors over which he had no control. Behavior modification techniques were totally unsuccessful in this case, because the behaviors are not voluntary and so the child cannot stop. The impulse to inflict injury in children with Lesch-Nyhan syndrome is an example of the definition of the term compulsion—namely, an irresistible impulse.

Children with Lesch-Nyhan syndrome also have trouble with gout and kidney stones because of the chemicals that accumulate in their bodies. These are painful and life-threatening complications of the disease. Medication is available to prevent the gout and kidney stones, but unfortunately there is no cure for the terrible compulsions associated with Lesch-Nyhan syndrome. It is important to make the diagnosis of Lesch-Nyhan syndrome as soon as possible, for several reasons. Once the diagnosis is established, proper precautions to avoid disfiguring self-mutilation (restraints and tooth removal) can be taken. Appropriate therapy can be initiated, taking into account the involuntary nature of the compulsions and destructive, aggressive behavior. Genetic counseling is also an important consideration for family members. Since this is an X-linked genetic disease, the mother is the carrier of the defective gene; this means that each of her sons will have a 50-50 chance of inheriting the defective gene and being afflicted with the disease, and each of her daughters will have a 50-50 chance of being carriers for the disease. Sisters of women with sons who have X-linked genetic diseases like Lesch-Nyhan syndrome have a 50-50 chance of being carriers, too, and genetic testing and counseling is advised. Genetic testing can determine if any woman is a carrier of Lesch-Nyhan syndrome. Prenatal diagnosis is available for Lesch-Nyhan syndrome.

There has been extensive research into the cause of Lesch-Nyhan syndrome. The protein responsible for causing Lesch-Nyhan syndrome has been purified and studied. The defective gene that causes Lesch-Nyhan syndrome has been cloned and studied extensively. We know the chemical ramifications of the enzyme deficiency, but we still haven't figured out how this defect causes this bizarre behavior.

Even more confusing is that, using genetic engineering techniques, mice have been produced with the exact enzyme deficiency as patients with Lesch-Nyhan syndrome, but these mice exhibit no evidence of bizarre behavior, self-mutilation, or mental dysfunction.

However, if normal rats are given large doses of caffeine (a chemical related to some of the chemicals that accumulate in the blood of patients with Lesch-Nyhan syndrome), they will begin to self-mutilate. This observation may be an important clue.

If we can discover why people with Lesch-Nyhan syndrome self-mutilate, this would have important implications in the study of chemical determinants of behavior.

Despite extensive research, there is still no treatment available to prevent the compulsions in these boys. For this and other reasons, Lesch-Nyhan syndrome may be the first genetic disease to be treated with gene replacement therapy. Calvin's parents have often told me that they would gladly submit him to experimental treatment if there was even a remote chance that the treatment would help Calvin's problems.

Any child with mental dysfunction or unusual behavior patterns or spasticity who develops gout and/or a kidney stone should be evaluated for Lesch-Nyhan syndrome.

Self-Mutilation: Congenital Indifference to Pain

A recessive genetic disease, *congenital indifference to pain* causes the inability to detect and to respond appropriately to pain. Like children with Lesch-Nyhan syndrome, children with congenital indifference to pain may chew off the ends of their tongues and injure their lips. Unlike Lesch-Nyhan syndrome, however, the self-mutilation is not due to an irresistible compulsion, but results from the inability of these children to experience pain as an unpleasant sensation. Patients with congenital indifference to pain have none of the usual physiologic reactions to pain such as increase in heart rate, breathing rate, or blood pressure. They do not withdraw from painful stimuli such as a pinprick or a burn. Bone deformities can develop in these children because they are unaware of broken bones.

Individuals with congenital indifference to pain are of normal intelligence and can be taught how to avoid injuring themselves. Because these children are often stigmatized by their "bizarre" behaviors in response to pain, it is important to make the diagnosis, even though they may learn how to compensate on their own.

Williams Syndrome: The Cocktail Party
Personality

Williams syndrome is a multiple malformation syndrome whose cause is unknown. Some scientists classify Williams syndrome as a genetic disease, but it does not follow classic inheritance patterns of autosomal dominant, recessive, or X-linked diseases. Williams syndrome seems to have a genetic component, so it belongs in the category of diseases with a genetic influence. Williams syndrome can cause low birth weight, peculiar-looking face, heart problems, short stature, and a characteristic star-like pattern in the iris (colored portion) of the eyes. In the newborn period, children with Williams syndrome may have elevations of calcium in their blood that normalize on their own by six months of age. Calcium levels are not routinely checked in well newborns, so most children diagnosed with Williams syndrome have no history of calcium elevations. Infants and children with Wiliams syndrome often have hoarse cries and hoarse voices.

Children with Williams syndrome are usually mentally retarded and delayed in developing motor skills. Individuals with Williams syndrome differ in one unusual respect from other retarded persons: they possess good social skills. Most mentally retarded children and adults have difficulty in social situations, while individuals with Williams syndrome are usually extremely skilled in making conversation. They are loquacious and socially adept, even though they are mentally retarded. This has led to the phrase "cocktail party personality" to describe people with Williams syndrome.

It is quite remarkable to see an individual with an IQ of 69 (in the mentally retarded range) at ease in adult social situations. I tell parents of these children that what their children say will not be profound, but they will say it very well.

There is no medical treatment for children with Williams syndrome. However, knowing the diagnosis and that strengths will be in verbal communication can lead to an educational program with these strengths in mind.

Any child with mental handicap and congenital heart disease, elevated calcium levels in the newborn period, a hoarse voice, or a "cocktail party personality" should be evaluated by a geneticist for the possibility of Williams syndrome.

Cornelia de Lange Syndrome: Aggressive or Autistic Behavior

Named after the scientist who discovered this disease, *Cornelia de Lange* syndrome is a multiple malformation syndrome whose cause is unknown. Like Williams syndrome (above), Cornelia de Lange syndrome has a genetic component but does not follow the strict inheritance patterns of a true genetic disease. In Cornelia de Lange syndrome, the genetic influence is inferred from the higher recurrence rate (3%) of affected children for parents of a previous child with this disorder.

Cornelia de Lange syndrome is recognized by a characteristic facial appearance including bushy eyebrows that meet in the middle of the forehead (medical term, synophrys), and unusually formed lips and skull. Most children with Cornelia de Lange syndrome become quite hairy after infancy (hirsutism), all are of short stature, and all are mentally retarded.

The mental dysfunction in children with Cornelia de
Lange syndrome is quite stereotyped. As infants their physical activity is sluggish, their muscle tone is increased (tight
muscles), and they have a low-pitched cry that almost
sounds like growling. Most children with this disease develop extremely aggressive behavior toward others and
sometimes themselves and use repetitive motions for self-
stimulation and calming. This cluster of behaviors can lead
to an incorrect diagnosis of infantile autism.

Behavior modification techniques are not helpful in
treating the aggressive or repetitive behaviors. As in Lesch-
Nyhan syndrome, these behaviors seem to be the result
of irresistible impulses. Once the diagnosis is made and
the involuntary nature of the aggressive behavior is understood, an appropriate educational placement can be
made.

There is no prenatal diagnosis available for Cornelia
de Lange syndrome.

Wilson's Disease: Psychosis and Mental Illness

Wilson's Disease is a recessive genetic disease in which
the body is unable to handle the mineral copper. Wilson's
disease can cause liver damage, mental disturbance, or
both. The mental disturbances affect the center of the
brain that involves coordination and may also cause symptoms resembling psychiatric disturbances. The psychiatric
symptoms can include schizophrenia, adolescent adjust-
ment problem, bizarre behavior, anxiety neurosis, mania,
depression, hysteria, and psychosis. Any adolescent who

has any of these psychiatric symptoms in addition to any neurological symptoms such as hand tremor or lack of coordination should be evaluated for the possibility of Wilson's disease *immediately.* This is because Wilson's disease is treatable!

If Wilson's disease is untreated, copper deposits form in the irises of the eye, creating a rust-colored ring at the border between the whites of the eye and the iris. This is called a Kaiser-Fleisher ring and indicates that the patient probably has Wilson's disease. This ring may not be present, or may be difficult to see early in the disease, however, so its absence should not prevent a further evaluation for the presence of Wilson's disease. Testing for Wilson's disease is quite difficult and requires a referral to a genetic specialist. The evaluation for Wilson's disease includes a medical examination, blood tests (copper and ceruloplasm), and an eye examination by an ophthalmologist (to look for the beginnings of a Kaiser-Fleisher ring). A liver biopsy may be necessary to establish the diagnosis.

It is important to consider the possibility of Wilson's disease, because Wilson's disease can be treated with medicine. Treatment can reverse some of the mental symptoms, and can prevent the eventual death of the patient from liver disease or neurological deterioration. In addition, it is important to know that a psychiatric patient has Wilson's disease, because the standard medications usually used for treating psychosis actually make the symptoms of individuals with Wilson's disease worse. It has been suggested that all adolescents admitted to inpatient psychiatric facilities be screened for Wilson's disease.

Premature Aging

There are several different genetic diseases that cause premature aging and senility in children. Often children with these disorders resemble elderly people by the time they are 6–16 years old. Their skin becomes dry and wrinkled, their walking becomes slow and labored, and they begin to be forgetful and develop senility before adolescence. The grown-up appearance of these child-sized people gave one of these diseases the name *leprechaunism*. These children may have been the model for the first legends of leprechauns. It is important to recognize such children because they are at a very high risk of developing cancer and must be followed closely. The diseases of premature aging include *progeria*, *Bloom's syndrome*, and *leprechaunism*.

Porphyria: Vampire Disease

There seems little doubt that legends about vampires evolved because of families with a genetic dominant disease called *porphyria*. (See also Chapters 7 and 10.) People with porphyria can have extremely sensitive skin that blisters when exposed even briefly to sunlight. People afflicted with porphyria are often anemic (have low blood counts) and develop cravings for red meat and other "bloody" foods containing iron; iron helps the body make more blood cells. Affected individuals are also prone to episodes of excruciating abdominal pain that can be associated with violent, uncontrollable impulses or with other symptoms of mental illness. Seizures can also occur during these episodes.

Porphyria is an autosomal dominant genetic disease, so each child of an affected parent has a 50-50 chance of having the disease. Thus, there are families with several generations of affected individuals who go outdoors only at night to avoid exposing their skin to damaging sunlight, have cravings for blood-containing foods, and are prone to fits of pain, and erratic, perhaps violent behavior. It is easy to imagine how vampire legends might have started in an ignorant society observing such a family.

Another aspect of porphyria is that the urine of individuals can turn red when exposed to heat or sunlight (see Chapter 7). I don't know if this contributed to the vampire legend, but it can certainly suggest the diagnosis of porphyria to an astute clinician.

There are several different kinds of porphyrias. The symptoms in any individual will vary according to the type of porphyria. Some affected individuals will have only intermittent abdominal pain without skin sensitivity or mental disturbance. Any individual who complains of intermittent abdominal pain and has any sort of behavioral or mental disturbance should be evaluated for porphyria. Blood and urine tests can be performed to determine if an individual has porphyria.

Tics and Attention Deficit Disorder—
Tourette's Syndrome

Tourette's syndrome is a fascinating dominant genetic disease in which affected children have various forms of learning disabilities (especially attention deficit disorder) in addition to tics. The tics may be either muscular, usually involving facial muscles, or can be vocal, when the child suddenly utters unusual sounds. Swearing, barking like a dog, or other animal noises have been described in children with Tourette's syndrome. Sometimes affected children may simply blurt out single syllables or staccato barrages of sound.

Tourette's syndrome is a genetic dominant disease, so that evidence of tics and learning problems in a parent suggests evaluation for Tourette's in a child with learning disabilities. It is important to make the diagnosis of Tourette's syndrome because effective medication regimens are available to treat these children.

Lead Poisoning: Irritability, Loss of Memory, Clumsiness

Although less of a problem currently than it was 20 years ago, *lead poisoning* continues to pose a health hazard, especially to children living in the inner cities. Crumbling exterior and old interior paint combine with leaded exhaust emissions to contaminate buildings and the dirt found in playgrounds near highways. Lead exposure can also come from home remodeling or furniture restoring when lead-based paint is sanded or scraped. Children are much more susceptible to the damaging affects of lead than adults. Nausea, headache, irritability, and clumsiness are all symptoms of lead poisoning. A simple blood test called FEP (free erythrocyte protoporphyrin) can determine whether or not a child is suffering from lead poisoning.

The prompt recognition and diagnosis of lead poisoning is essential because, if left untreated, lead poisoning can lead to permanent brain damage. If recognized, children can be treated with special medicines (called chelators) to remove the lead from the body.

Obesity and Mental Retardation

There are several birth defect syndromes that result in obesity and mental deficiency. The most common is a multiple malformation syndrome known as *Prader-Willi syndrome*. Prader-Willi syndrome is caused by a small deletion in one chromosome. Children with Prader-Willi syndrome can have moderate to severe mental retardation, short stature, obesity beginning in infancy, fair hair and complexion, poor muscle tone, small hands and feet, and undescended testicles in boys. It is important to keep in mind that in Prader-Willi syndrome, as in other multiple malformation syndromes, a child may not have all of the features listed above and still have the disease.

There are several other multiple malformation syndromes that cause mental retardation and obesity. These include *Laurence-Moon-Bardet-Biedl syndrome, Börjeson-Forssman-Lehmann syndrome, Carpenter's syndrome, Cohen syndrome,* and *Killian/Teschler-Nicola syndrome.* A geneticist will be able to determine if a particular child has one of these syndromes. Since some of these disorders are genetic diseases, it is important to make the diagnosis so that parents can be counseled with respect to recurrence risk.

Masklike Face

There are some multiple malformation syndromes that affect facial nerves and muscles and cause the child's facial expression to remain constant, as if the child is wearing a mask. It is very difficult to work with such a child because he has no way of registering emotions using facial expressions. Such a child should be referred for medical evaluation to determine the exact cause of this phenomenon. There are four disorders capable of causing masklike faces: *Facio-auriculo-vertebral syndrome, Freeman Sheldon syndrome, Schwartz syndrome,* and *Steinert muscular dystrophy.*

The disorders discussed thus far in this chapter produce stereotyped behavior in affected individuals. In the disorders discussed below, the disease creates a *predisposition* toward a particular mental problem, but affected individuals may not suffer from them.

Immature Behavior: XXX Syndrome

Girls with an extra sex chromosome may have problems with speech, coordination, and immature behavior. After puberty, these girls tend to be tall. This constellation of signs suggests the need for a chromosomal evaluation. Although there is no specific medical treatment for XXX girls, the diagnosis identifies the etiology of their mental dysfunction.

Fragile X Syndrome: Autisticlike Behavior

The Fragile X syndrome is an X-linked genetic disease that affects mostly boys. A special blood test can unequivocally establish the diagnosis. Many children with Fragile X Syndrome have hyperactivelike behavior patterns that are sometimes referred to as "pervasive motor activity." Children with this behavior pattern are incessantly moving and fidgeting. Because of this incessant activity in combination with mental dysfunction (see Chapter 6), many children with Fragile X Syndrome have actually been diagnosed as having infantile autism, a severe disorder in which children are unable to interact with others. Twenty percent of all individuals with the Fragile X syndrome have been previously diagnosed as having infantile autism.

I saw a seven-year-old boy in consultation who had been referred to a psychiatrist colleague of mine with the diagnosis of infantile autism. After examining the boy, the psychiatrist was convinced that the child was not autistic, because he was able to make and briefly hold eye contact and was able to relate to his mother, behaviors that truly autistic children usually cannot do. Fragile X testing revealed that this child does have the Fragile X syndrome.

Most children with the Fragile X syndrome do not have behavior abnormalities severe enough to be classified autistic however. Many are mentally retarded or learning disabled without hyperactive components (the fidgeting and continuous movement). Some will have combinations of mental and behavior dysfunction. Somehow the genetic abnormality combines with the child's own personality and his environment to cause the aberrant behavior. We could conclude that having Fragile X syndrome predisposes development of autisticlike behavior, but does not, in and of itself, cause such behavior.

Therefore mental retardation, learning disability, and behavior disorder can all be caused by the Fragile X syndrome (see Chapter 6).

Klinefelter's Syndrome and XYY Syndrome

Other examples of genetic predisposition to behavioral problems are Klinefelter's syndrome and XYY syndrome. These disorders were discussed in detail in Chapter 6. Klinefelter's syndrome and XYY syndrome are genetic diseases caused by the presence of an extra sex chromosome, either an extra X or an extra Y chromosome. The diagnosis of these disorders can be established by a blood test (karyotype) that analyzes and individual's chromosomes.

As discussed in Chapter 6, men with Klinefelter's syndrome are at a 10 times higher risk of developing mental illness than the general population. However, 98 out of every 100 men with Klinefelter's syndrome will not ever have mental illness.

Summary

This chapter has identified genetic and nongenetic diseases that lead to stereotyped behavior patterns. Any child demonstrating one of these behavior patterns should have a genetic evaluation.

Chapter 9

Diseases Causing Loss of Developmental Milestones

Some diseases can cause sudden or gradual mental deterioration. Children with these diseases progressively lose their physical and intellectual abilities, and this is called loss of developmental milestones. *Any child who has either an unexplained loss of developmental milestones, deterioration of physical performance, or intellectual deterioration should have a medical evaluation immediately.*

It is important to differentiate between true loss of developmental milestones and regression. Emotional, physical, and social stresses may cause children to "regress." Regression in this sense refers to returning to a less developmentally advanced stage. Depending on the age when regression occurs, regression can take the form of loss of toilet training skills, sleep disorders, "clinginess," or school anxiety. In extreme instances a child may stop speaking. Usually, but not always, gross and fine motor skills and intellectual skills remain intact.

The mental deterioration of children is often so gradual that parents and teachers miss it. Sometimes relatives
who haven't seen the child for several months will be the
first to notice that deterioration has taken place.

When evaluating a child for mental deterioration it
is important to attempt to identify any *new* stresses in
the life of the child to explain his regression. If a major
stress factor such as death of a parent, divorce, or a classroom change is identified, regression is likely to be the
cause of the child's dysfunction. Even if no stress factor
can be identified, it is possible that a child's loss of abilities is due to regression and not a true loss of milestones.
The type of skills lost is also important. A child who loses
the ability to hop or hold a pencil is at a higher risk for
having a true loss of milestones than a child who begins
to have urinary accidents. However, this distinction is not
absolute. Sometimes it is only after several months or
years of observation that suspicions of physical disease
arise.

One such child was Larry, who was described in
Chapter 7. Larry had normal mental function at age 12
but became progressively mentally handicapped. Larry's
problems began around the time his parents divorced and
his abilities progressively deteriorated each year after that.
Initially Larry's poor school performance was attributed
to the psychological trauma surrounding his parents' divorce.

The progression of his school photos documented as
no textbook ever could the true pattern of "loss of milestones." Testing revealed that Larry has a degenerative genetic disease called metachromatic leukodystrophy (see
below). Unfortunately there is no cure or treatment for
this disease. Since Larry's mother is divorced and not plan-

ning to have future children, genetic counseling was not an issue. Since this disease is recessive, each child of Larry's mother and father would have a 25% risk of having the disease.

The proper diagnosis of metachromatic leukodystrophy was important for this family. We were able to give Larry's mother an accurate (if dismal) prognosis for her son, namely that his regression would continue until an early death. We also demonstrated that her divorce was not the cause of Larry's problems. This information lifted a tremendous burden of guilt from her shoulders.

As soon as you suspect that a child has suffered a true loss of developmental milestones, the appropriate initial referral is to a pediatric neurologist. The neurologist will assess the current functioning of the brain, nerves, and muscles, and may be able to establish a diagnosis for the child, such as a brain tumor or degenerative neurological disease such as *Huntington's chorea*. If the neurologist is unable to establish a diagnosis, a referral to a biochemical geneticist is necessary. The geneticist can evaluate the individual for the presence of genetic diseases that may be the cause of the neurological deterioration.

Although the majority of this chapter deals with genetic causes of loss of developmental milestones, there are a few nongenetic causes of mental deterioration that are important to consider.

Head trauma, near-drowning, and *acute brain infections* such as *meningitis* or *encephalitis* are capable of causing brain damage. These conditions cause injury at the time of the trauma or infection. Milestones can be lost immediately after the episode, but not months or years later.

Less easy to detect, however, is a disease known as SSPE (subacute sclerosing panencephalitis). This is an insidious disease caused by a viral infection of the brain and causes progressive brain damage over a period of months to years. There is no cure for SSPE at this time. Children with SSPE may have no symptoms of infection. Loss of milestones, and deterioration of intellectual and motor skills, may be the only symptoms of SSPE. These changes may be quite gradual and subtle. A neurologist will be able to confirm the diagnosis of SSPE.

Lead and mercury poisonings may also lead to mental deterioration. Irritability, headaches, and clumsiness are usually present in a child with lead or mercury poisoning (see Chapter 8).

Brain tumors, strokes, and aneurysms are rare, but do occur in children. These diseases can be diagnosed by a neurologist using special X rays of the brain called CT (computerized tomography) scans or MRI (magnetic resonance imaging) scans.

Lysosomal Storage Diseases

Loss of developmental milestones is characteristic in children with one of several diseases collectively known as *lysosomal storage diseases.* Most of the lysosomal storage diseases are autosomal recessive which means that no one in either parent's family will have had the disease. The disease only occurs when two carriers have children. Parents who have one child with a lysosomal storage disease have a 25% risk of each subsequent child also having the disorder.

A few of the lysosomal storage diseases are X-linked, which means there may be a family history of a grandfather, maternal uncle, or male cousin affected. (For more information regarding the lysosomal storage diseases see Scriver et al., 1989.)

Lysosomes are the garbage disposers of cells. Each cell contains several lysosomes. All areas of the body are continually regenerated. Old material is removed and new material is deposited to keep our bodies supple and functional. The old, decayed material is taken into cells and partitioned into the lysosomes. The lysosomes are self-contained digestive units containing scores of enzymes to digest every conceivable chemical bond made in nature. Like the insides of our stomachs, the inside of the lysosome is extremely acidic.

Once the waste products have entered the lysosomes, the acid and enzymes act to completely digest the insoluble (not dissolvable in water) products into nontoxic soluble molecules that can be reused by the cells to make new materials, or can pass through the blood for eventual excretion by the kidney into urine, or by the liver into stool.

In lysosomal storage diseases, one or more of the enzymes responsible for digesting a particular type of chemical bond is defective. For example the lysosomal storage disease known as Tay-Sachs disease results from a deficiency of an enzyme called hexosaminidase A. This enzyme is responsible for digesting a very large complex molecule known as GM_2 ganglioside, a substance found in high concentrations in the brain.

Like most other lysosomal diseases, Tay-Sachs disease is autosomal recessive, so both parents of an affected child are carriers for the disease. The carrier parents have one normal gene and one defective gene. Therefore the lysosomes of the parents contain about half of the active enzyme than noncarriers.

Carriers of Tay-Sachs disease have no symptoms. This

is because their lysosomes can function perfectly well with only half the usual amount of enzyme. This is analogous to adding one half cup of laundry detergent instead of a full cup to the wash—the clothes still get clean. Actually, for most enzymes in our body, only 20% of normal activity is sufficient to insure a completely healthy individual. This built-in safety factor insures that carriers for genetic diseases will not suffer any consequences from their genetic makeup.

Blood tests can be performed to determine if individuals are carriers for Tay-Sachs disease. The tests measure the levels of hexosaminidase A. Since there is a high frequency of carriers for Tay-Sachs disease in the Ashkenazic Jewish population (about 1 in 30 are carriers), carrier detection testing for Tay-Sachs disease is highly recommended for members of this group before pregnancy.

If two carriers for Tay-Sachs disease have children together, each child has a 25% risk of inheriting the defective gene from both parents and having Tay-Sach's disease. The lysosomes of a child with Tay-Sachs disease have virtually no active hexosaminidase A. Because of this, lysosomes from these patients are totally unable to digest the large molecules of GM_2 ganglioside. Since this material is primarily found in the brain, brain cells are damaged most severely. The cells take up the old GM_2 ganglioside and partition it into lysosomes for digestion and removal. But the lysosomes of a patient with Tay-Sachs disease are totally incapable of digesting the material. The GM_2 ganglioside continues to accumulate inside the cell's lysosomes and the lysosomes swell in size because they are unable to rid themselves of the waste material. Like a stream that has been dammed, the lysosomes continue to grow in size until the entire cell is filled with these dysfunctional, swollen lysosomes. Eventually the cells become so bloated with lysosomes that they can no longer maintain the necessary life-supporting functions, and the cells die.

The brain contains the largest concentration of GM_2 ganglioside, so it is the brain cells of a child with Tay-Sachs disease that are primarily affected. The body can never make new brain cells after birth, so there is no way to replace the dead brain cells in a child with Tay-Sachs disease. The continual death of brain cells leads to progressive mental deterioration and death prior to the age of six years. Death occurs because the brain becomes unable to control the basic functions of breathing and heartbeat regulation.

The curve marked "Profound loss" on page 9 is representative of a typical child with Tay-Sachs disease. These children appear completely normal at birth because it takes several months for the lysosomes to become filled with debris. Children with Tay-Sachs disease usually develop normally for the first 6 months of life. Sometime between 6 months and 1 year of life, mental dysfunction becomes noticeable, when brain cells begin to die. First, there is an apparent slowing of development, and then loss of milestones occurs. As the child's condition continues to deteriorate he becomes blind, vegetative, and finally dies.

There is no cure for Tay-Sachs disease, or for any of the lysosomal storage diseases. Carrier screening and prenatal diagnosis can prevent the birth of children with Tay-Sachs disease.

The diagnosis of a lysosomal storage disease establishes an accurate prognosis and permits genetic counseling for the parents and siblings who are at risk of having other affected children.

Tay-Sachs disease is only one of several lysosomal storage diseases. Each disorder has its own characteristic symptoms and signs. Each disease has its own enzyme defect leading to the inability to digest a particular body waste product. The symptoms of each disease depend on the nature of the material and where it is found in the body. For example, GM_2 ganglioside is found primarily in brain, so children with Tay-Sachs have mental deterioration as their primary symptom.

Dermatan and heparan sulfate, the substances that cannot be digested in the disease known as *Hurler's disease*, are found in skin, tendons, joints, and bones, in addition to the brain. Children with Hurler's disease suffer from stiff joints, and have very peculiar bone structure in addition to their mental dysfunction. Hunter disease (Chapter 7) is another example of a lysosomal storage disease leading to peculiar-looking facial appearance. As noted, distinctive facial appearance led to the common name for these syndromes, "gargoylism."

It is important to note that all of the lysosomal storage diseases are *progressive diseases*. Almost always, newborns and infants look and act healthy and normal. Physical and mental symptoms may progress insidiously in some of the lysosomal storage diseases.

One of the children I saw at the Laremont School was a six-year-old boy who appeared to have one of the lysosomal storage diseases. I noticed his "gargoyle" appearance from 100 feet away. When I examined him he was unable to raise his hands above his head, a classic symptom of the lysosomal storage disease that causes the gargoyle-like appearance known as Hunter's disease (see Chapter 7). The exact diagnosis could be confirmed with a blood and urine test. The physical features characteristic of several of the lysosomal storage diseases become more obvious as the child grows. This child's features probably were not as pronounced at birth and when he was last evaluated medically, or the diagnosis would have been made at that time.

The diagnosis of children with lysosomal storage diseases is complicated not only by the insidious onset of several of these disorders, but by the variability of symptoms and times of onset. This variability may be due to differences in the amount of enzyme activity; some children have absolutely no enzyme activity whereas others may have between 1–10 percent of normal activity. This "residual activity" can produce a milder form of the disease.

Table 9 shows the symptoms of children with various lysosomal storage diseases. Except where noted, all these disorders cause neurological dysfunction. Although loss of developmental milestones is the most common symptom for these children, they may be diagnosed as mildly or moderately retarded or developmentally delayed. The diagnosis of a lysosomal storage disease is made by biochemical testing of the child's urine and/or blood. These tests are usually performed by biochemical geneticist.

Any child suspected of having a lysosomal storage disease should be referred to a geneticist for evaluation.

There are other genetic diseases, in addition to the lysosomal storage diseases, that can cause loss of developmental milestones.

Stroke—Homocystinuria

Homocystinuria is a genetic disease causing a biochemical imbalance in the blood of affected children. Children

Table 9. Physical Symptoms of
Children with Lysosomal
Storage Diseases

Loss of developmental milestones
Coarse facial appearance
Coarse hair
General hairiness (hirsutism)
Brittle hair
Thick skin
Coarse skin
Poor dentition, multiple cavities
Joint stiffness (including spine)
Poor vision
Poor coordination
Seizures
Cataracts
Cloudy corneas
Glaucoma
Short stature
Short neck
Abnormal bone X rays
Unusual facial appearance not resembling
    parents or siblings in nonadopted
    children
Limitation of joint movement (especially
    in the shoulders—see if the child
    can grasp his hands over his head)
Short neck or stiff spine
Unusual body proportions

with homocystinuria have two kinds of mental dysfunction. Most children with homocystinuria are mentally retarded. They may also suffer strokes that cause a loss of milestones. Strokes are quite rare in childhood. Any child who is suspected of having a stroke should be evaluated immediately for homocystinuria by a biochemical geneticist.

Table 10. Features
of Homocystinuria

Long arms and legs
    with respect to
    the body
Flat feet
Stiff joints
Nearsightedness
Lens dislocations
Mental retardation
Learning disability
Stroke

It is crucial to make the diagnosis of homocystinuria because most of the time it is treatable. In about half the cases of homocystinuria, megadoses of pyridoxine (vitamin B_6) will correct the biochemical imbalance in the blood. If vitamin therapy is unsuccessful, another drug called betaine is often successful in treating the biochemical imbalance. Correcting the biochemical imbalance in these children often results in an improvement in mental functioning and can prevent future strokes from occurring.

Homocystinuria also affects the skeletal system. Children with homocystinuria often have long arms and legs in proportion to their bodies (called marfanoid body proportions). They can also have stiff joints. Children with homocystinuria are nearsighted and sometimes, later in life, the lenses in their eyes may become dislodged (lens dislocations).

All children who have mental dysfunction in combination with any of the features listed in Table 10 should be evaluated by a biochemical geneticist.

Chapter 10

Inborn Errors of Metabolism

This chapter discusses a group of several hundred disorders collectively known as *inborn errors of metabolism* or *inherited metabolic diseases*. All of these disorders are genetic (hence the term inherited) and they all involve defects in the body's performance of one or more of the thousands of chemical reactions necessary for proper bodily function. The lysosomal storage diseases, discussed in Chapter 9, are a subclass of these disorders. Children with inherited metabolic diseases inherit defective genes that are responsible for producing a single enzyme. Each enzyme performs a particular chemical reaction in the body. The importance of the chemical reaction to the body determines the severity of the illness and which systems (i.e., brain, muscles, kidneys) are primarily affected.

Clinical Variability in Inherited Metabolic Disease

One of the most intriguing aspects of treating children with inherited metabolic disease is the variability of symptoms in children with the same disease. Even siblings with the same genetic disease can have tremendous variability in the severity of their illness. A good example of this variability is illustrated by two children in the same family with an inherited metabolic disease called *isovaleric acidemia* (see also Chapter 6). This disease is caused when a child inherits a defective recessive gene from both parents for the enzyme that digests certain amino acids contained in all proteins.

The firstborn child of this couple had died in the newborn period. He appeared completely normal at birth, but on the third day of life became listless and lapsed into coma. He was rushed to a hospital, where he was given antibiotics and placed on IV fluids. He remained in coma for three days and then regained consciousness.

It was assumed that an infection had caused the problem, although none of the cultures were positive. Three days after discharge from the hospital, his parents found him unconscious in his crib. They again rushed him to the hospital, where he died after three days of coma. No cause was found for the baby's death. The death certificate attributed the cause of death to sudden infant death syndrome. Eighteen months later the parents had their second child, a girl. This girl did very well in infancy and, although her neurological development was slow, her parents had no suspicion that anything was wrong. When she was three and a half years old, on Thanksgiving night, she began vomiting after the meal. She was very sleepy, so her parents put her to bed, assuming that overstimulation was the cause of her problem.

The following morning, she continued to vomit and

was extremely difficult to awaken. She was taken to a hospital, where she was treated for dehydration with intravenous fluids. She finally perked up after three days. Over the next 18 months, she had three similar episodes, and all were treated in the same manner. During her fifth episode, however, she did not wake up after seven days of therapy, so she was transferred to my care.

Biochemical testing revealed that she had isovaleric acidemia. Appropriate treatments with medications and a low protein diet were initiated. She woke up and has not had any further episodes. Upon entering school, however, a learning disability involving visual-perceptual processing and attention deficit disorder were identified, probably the result of brain damage from her episodes of sleepiness.

In reviewing the records of her brother who died in infancy, it seemed probable that he, too, had isovaleric acidemia. Why was the brother affected so much more severely than the sister? We don't know. The sister has the intermittent form of isovaleric acidemia, and her brother probably had the neonatal form of isovaleric acidemia. Both children must have inherited the *identical* defective genes (one from each parent), and yet one died in the newborn period and the other was three years of age before symptoms developed.

Clinical variability occurs to a greater or lesser extent in all inherited metabolic diseases. The same disease can cause mental retardation in some children and learning disability in others. That is why the following section does not discriminate between those disorders that can cause mental retardation and those that cause learning disabilities.

Most inherited metabolic diseases are capable of causing mental dysfunction. This section describes some general features of inborn errors of metabolism and then discusses in more detail certain diseases that are of particular relevance to mental dysfunction.

Phenylketonuria (PKU) is an inherited metabolic disease. As mentioned in Chapter 7, the successful treatment of PKU with specially designed low protein diets was the first successful prevention of mental retardation. In PKU, the body is unable to digest the amino acid phenylalanine, a component of all naturally occurring protein. When infants with phenylketonuria eat protein, toxic products build up in their blood because they cannot digest the amino acid phenylanine. This causes irreversible brain damage. Studies show that for every month a child with PKU is untreated, 5 IQ points will be lost. If the disease remains untreated, the child will become profoundly retarded and be nearly vegetative by the end of the second year of life.

Fortunately, an extremely restrictive low-protein diet is an effective treatment for PKU. This diet requires close medical supervision to assure sufficient nutrition.

In infancy, the cornerstone of PKU diets are synthetic formulas from which the phenylalanine has been removed. After infancy, special low-protein diets are designed by nutrition experts. Children with PKU who are successfully treated with this special diet can have completely normal intelligence. The diet must be continued throughout life to obtain optimal results.

Since untreated PKU causes irreversible brain damage, it is important to diagnose and begin treatment of PKU in the newborn period. Hospitals in the United States now routinely screen all newborns for the presence of PKU and other treatable causes of mental retardation. Two to three days after birth, the heel of the infant is pricked, and spots of blood are placed on special cards containing a special paper. These "heel stick blood spots" are then sent to laboratories where they are analyzed for a variety of diseases. If the screening test indicates a possibility of PKU, a special blood test is performed to confirm the diagnosis.

All 50 states and the District of Columbia have newborn screening programs for PKU and another treatable cause of mental retardation called *congenital hypothyroidism* (low thyroid). In some states the screening is mandatory and in other states it is voluntary. Sometimes a child may not be tested because the parents refuse the test in states where the testing is voluntary or the baby was not born in a hospital. Even children who are tested in newborn screening programs can "slip through the cracks." The laboratory may make a mistake in the analysis, or the specimen card may be mislabeled. The longer the delay in the diagnosis of PKU, the greater permanent brain damage will occur, so it is important to consider this diagnosis in any infant with poor development, especially if the child has a fair complexion, another symptom of PKU. It is tragic to miss diagnosing a child with PKU or congenital hypothyroidism.

Congenital hypothyroidism is the result of a failure of the thyroid gland to make enough thyroid hormone. If left untreated, this disease leads to severe mental retardation and stunted growth. The medical term for an untreated individual with congenital hypothyroidism is "cretin." Once diagnosed, congenital hypothyroidism is treated by giving replacement thyroid hormone by mouth.

Even though all newborn screening programs test for congenital hypothyroidism, they may not detect all cases of children with hypothyroidism due to the variability in laboratory methods used to detect the disease and the existence of different types of hypothyroidism, some of which cannot be detected by currently available techniques. Therefore, it is probable that the diagnosis of some children with congenital hypothyroidism will be missed by newborn screening programs. The symptoms of congenital hypothyroidism include developmental delay, mental retardation, extremely short stature, and delayed closure of the fontanelles (soft spots in the head). The diagnosis of congenital hypothyroidism requires a special blood test.

There are four other disorders in the category of inborn errors of metabolism that cause *preventable mental retardation*. These diseases are galactosemia, biotinidase deficiency, congenital adrenal hyperplasia and homocystinuria, and are discussed below.

In some states, newborn screening programs include testing for these diseases. Since these diseases are preventable causes of mental retardation it is crucial to recognize the earliest signs and symptoms of these disorders. Since newborn screening tests are not established for them in all states, and many children who may have these diseases were born before the development of the test, children who show symptoms of these diseases should be promptly referred to a geneticist for evaluation.

If you suspect that a child may have one of these diseases, even if newborn screening was performed, I recommend that he be tested using the specific blood tests and not just the screening tests. If the test needs to be repeated, in most cases it will be free of charge. No test is infallible, especially when millions are done each year. If there is any doubt, repeat the test.

Children with *galactosemia* have an inability to digest the sugar present in cows' milk and breast milk. When infants with galactosemia are breast fed or given a commercial cows' milk-based formula, they develop jaundice (yellow skin), vomit frequently after feedings, and can become developmentally delayed. If the babies are changed to soy-based formula (such as Isomil or Prosobee) that do not contain milk sugar, they may not be obviously ill. Intermittent vomiting and developmental delay may be their only symptoms. Children with galactosemia are also prone to developing life-threatening infections in infancy, especially by a bacteria known as *E. coli*. Any child with a history of *E. coli* sepsis (blood infection) should be tested for galactosemia. Urine and blood tests can establish the diagnosis of galactosemia.

Biotinidase deficiency is a fascinating disorder. It is one form of a more general disease known as *multiple carboxylase deficiency*. Children with biotinidase deficiency and other forms of multiple carboxylase deficiency are unable to utilize properly the B-complex vitamin known as biotin. Like Marie in Chapter 3, affected children have developmental delay and poor coordination. Later in life, episodes of vomiting may develop. Some children with multiple carboxylase deficiency are very ill in infancy while other children's symptoms begin later in life and can be quite subtle. Some children with biotinidase deficiency have only a subtle learning disability. Seizures, mental retardation, and clumsiness can also be part of this disorder. Physical signs, such as recurrent yeast infections of the skin (candidiasis) and hair loss (alopecia) can also accompany multiple carboxylase deficiency.

It is very important to make the diagnosis of multiple carboxylase deficiency because children can be successfully treated with large doses (megadoses) of the vitamin biotin. In almost all cases, the biotin treatment *completely* eliminates and can sometimes even reverse the mental and physical dysfunction.

Biotin treatment of children with multiple carboxylase deficiency can be miraculous, like a cure in a revival meeting. Children who have been unable to stand or walk, can begin walking in a few weeks. Children who had frequent uncontrolled seizures can suddenly stop having seizures. The diagnosis of biotinidase deficiency can be made by a blood test. The diagnoses of other forms of multiple carboxylase deficiency are more difficult to make and require specialized tests.

Other Inherited Metabolic Diseases That Can Cause Mental Retardation or Learning Disability

There are over 200 different inherited metabolic diseases. Most of them are capable of causing mental dysfunction. This section begins with a discussion of some general symptoms that suggest the presence of inherited metabolic disease. Subsequently, some treatable disorders of particular interest to a discussion of learning disability are described.

Vomiting without Diarrhea

Children with certain forms of inherited metabolic disease (urea cycle defects and organic acidemias) suffer from recurrent episodes of vomiting. The episodes are usually triggered by viral infections that cause fever. The combination of fever and vomiting is usually attributed to a gastroenteritis or a "stomach flu." These episodes differ from gastroenteritis because vomiting occurs without diarrhea (see Chapter 7). Sometimes, if the episode is severe enough, the vomiting is followed by lethargy or coma. Lethargy is extreme sleepiness to the point of being barely arousable. Coma is unresponsiveness to any stimulation.

Gastroenteritis is treated by placing the patient on a clear liquid diet that is very low in protein content. The low-protein diet is, coincidentally, one of the treatments for the biochemical problem. Therefore, children with inherited metabolic diseases usually recover in 2–7 days from their vomiting episodes.

Any child who has recurrent episodes of vomiting (usually unaccompanied by diarrhea) needs an evaluation for an inherited metabolic disease, especially if lethargic behavior or coma is a part of the pattern. Treating the disorder may prevent further brain damage from biochemical toxicity, allow improved brain functioning, eliminate or reduce significantly the number and severity of the episodes and, most importantly, may prevent potentially lethal complications. The diagnosis of such a disorder can also lead to genetic counseling for parents who can be informed of the recurrence risk for future children.

Unusual Food Preferences

Many children with inherited metabolic diseases are unable to digest certain kinds of foods. They may experience symptoms of nausea or other unpleasant feelings after eating foods containing a large amount of the offending substance (see Chapter 7).

Children with a disease known as *hereditary fructose intolerance* are unable to digest the sugar fructose properly. Fructose is contained in table sugar (sucrose). Sucrose contains two sugars, glucose and fructose, linked together. Fruits contain plain fructose. When children with hereditary fructose intolerance eat fruits or foods containing table sugar, they become hypoglycemic (low blood sugar). Hypoglycemia causes a myriad of symptoms including nausea, vomiting, diarrhea, and sweating, and can cause seizures and brain damage (see Chapter 7).

During infancy, children are unable to avoid and/or recognize which foods are harmful to them. Sometimes they simply refuse to eat enough food and will grow poorly. As they grow, however, they may eventually notice that some foods cause discomfort and learn to avoid these foods.

If left untreated, children with hereditary fructose intolerance will fail to thrive, have mental dysfunction, and eventually die of liver cirrhosis. If the diagnosis is made and the disease is treated by eliminating all fructose from the diet, any further damage can be prevented and the child can live a long and healthy life.

Children with other types of inherited metabolic disease may demonstrate *protein* avoidance rather than sugar avoidance. These children may eventually learn to avoid milk, eggs, and meats (see Chapter 7).

Any child with a mental handicap and an usual pattern of food avoidance should be evaluated for an inherited metabolic disease.

Unfortunately, not all children with inherited metabolic diseases learn to avoid harmful foods. Children with a disorder related to hereditary fructose intolerance called *fructose 1,6 diphophatase deficiency* have a similar inability to digest fructose, but seldom learn to avoid the sugar. Children with this disorder continue to eat sugar and suffer increasing brain damage because of low blood sugar.

Seizures after Prolonged Fasts

The human body has two ways of getting the sugar it needs to maintain itself. The first way is by eating foods containing sugar; the second is to manufacture it using the basic chemicals already in the body. "Normal" individuals can make sugar by digesting muscle protein in the body. This is important because after a long fast (more than 18 hours) the body must make new sugar in order to maintain safe blood sugar levels. The brain needs a continuing supply of sugar to function normally. Children with inherited metabolic diseases are unable to make sugar by digesting muscle protein, and they experience low blood sugar (clamminess, nervousness, seizures) after not eating. These diseases have been called "Saturday night syndrome" because seizures occur after the child goes without eating for more than 18 hours; children put to bed early on Saturday night when their parents go out who sleep late on Sunday morning go without eating longer than usual. These children often have seizures due to low blood sugar.

It is important to mention at this point that the most common times for a child with a seizure disorder to have a convulsion are upon wakening and upon falling asleep. A child who has a seizure *after not eating for over 18 hours* should be evaluated for an inherited metabolic disease.

Children who have repeated episodes of low blood sugar are continually suffering brain damage, so it is essential that the diagnosis be made as soon as possible. Treatment can be as simple as waking an infant or child in the night for an extra feeding or meal. Children who experience irritability, tremors, nausea, stomach cramps, sweating, or clammy skin before meals should be evaluated for inherited metabolic disease.

Unusual Odor to Urine, Sweat, or Stool

The chemicals that accumulate in some children with inherited metabolic disease have distinctive odors. These are listed in Chapter 7. If a child has mental dysfunction and parents or teachers notice an usual odor to their sweat, bodies, urine, or stools, a metabolic evaluation is needed.

Rapid and/or Deep Breathing

Some children with inherited metabolic disease have, intermittently, a buildup of acids in their bodies. In an attempt to neutralize this acid, the body tries to breathe out as much carbon dioxide as possible. This can cause the child to have particularly rapid or particularly deep breathing patterns. In infancy these episodes can be misdiagnosed as pneumonia or bronchiolitis, and the metabolic cause for these symptoms can missed.

An 18-month-old patient was brought to me for evaluation of developmental delay with failure to gain height. In examining his chart, I noticed that he had three previous hospital admissions for pneumonia. On each admission, routine laboratory analysis of his blood revealed a high acid content. These results had been attributed to his pneumonia. However, he actually has an inherited metabolic disease that caused intermittent buildup of acids and mimicked recurrent pneumonia. I placed him on medication to neutralize acids and his growth improved, he stopped having episodes of "pneumonia," and his developmental progress improved dramatically.

The evaluation for possible inherited metabolic disease is quite complex and can only be done by a specialist in biochemical genetics. The evaluation may involve hospitalizations for special testing protocols designed to unmask symptoms. The American Board of Medical Genetics has a certification procedure for specialists in biochemical genetics. A listing of board-certified biochemical geneticists in your area can be obtained from the American Society of Human Genetics, Rockville Pike, Maryland.

Peroxosomal Disorders

A recently described class of inherited metabolic diseases that can contribute to mental dysfunction are the *peroxosomal disorders.* Children with these disorders have poor muscle tone, developmental delay, dysfunction of the adrenal glands, peculiar-looking faces, and/or liver damage. A special blood test called plasma long chain fatty acid analysis is necessary to evaluate the child for a peroxosomal disorder. Since these are recently described disorders, it is unlikely that older children born before 1986 would have been tested for peroxosomal diseases in infancy.

Other inherited metabolic diseases capable of causing mental dysfunction have been described in detail in previous chapters. These include the porphyrias (Chapter 8), Wilson's disease (Chapter 8), and homocystinuria (Chapter 9).

Chapter 11

Physical Features Associated with Mental Dysfunction

This chapter identifies physical abnormalities associated with mental dysfunction. When one or more of these physical attributes are observable in a child, a genetic evaluation is needed.

The following is not an exhaustive list by any means. The entire book, *Smith's Recognizable Pattern of Human Malformations* (Jones, 1988), is devoted to cataloging physical features suggestive of genetic diseases or multiple malformation syndromes.

Table 11 below lists abnormal physical findings associated with various genetic diseases and multiple malformation syndromes. Any child who has mental deficiency and one of these problems should have a genetic evaluation. This section is adapted from *Recognizable Patterns of Human Malformations.*

Table 11. Physical Features Associated with
Genetic Diseases and Multiple Malformation
Syndromes

Blindness
Ear abnormalities including absent earlobes,
   malformed earlobes, and skin tags
Extreme nearsightedness
Poor muscle tone in infancy (hypotonia)
Increased muscle tone in infancy (hypertonia)
Deafness
Extreme hearing loss
Water on the brain (hydrocephalus)
Small head (microcephaly)
Large head (macrocephaly)
Premature closure of the bones in the skull
   (craniosynostosis)
Unusual-looking face (dysmorphic features)
Eyelid folds (inner epicanthal folds, outer
   epicanthal folds)
Eyes slanting up (up-slanting palpebral fissures)
Eyes slanting down (down-slanting palpebral
   fissures)
Drooping eyelids (ptosis)
Jerking eye movements (nystagmus)
Small eyeballs (microphthalmia)
Imperfections of the iris (iris coloboma)
Glaucoma
Cataracts
Eyebrows that meet in the middle of the face
   (synophrys)
Double row of eyelashes
Short chin (micrognathia)
Abnormal teeth
Cleft lip
Cleft palate
Cleft lip and cleft palate
Large, protruding tongue (macroglossia)
Teeth present at birth (neonatal teeth)

Table 11. (*Continued*)

Webbed neck
Extremely long fingers (arachnodactyly)
Short neck
Extra fingers and/or toes (polydactyly)
Webbed fingers and/or toes (syndactyly)
Extremely broad thumbs
Small hands and/or feet
Absence of thumb or very small thumb (thumb
    hypoplasia)
Limitation of joint motion
Club foot
Loose-jointed or double-jointed (hyperextensible
    joints)
Loose skin
Thick skin
Large birthmarks
Sensitivity to light (photophobia)
Frequent skin rashes
Hair loss (alopecia)
Sparse hair
Coarse hair
Heart defect (congenital heart disease)
Kidney abnormality
Abnormal genitals
Obesity
Accelerated growth
Arms and/or legs of differing lengths (extremity
    asymmetry)
Short stature

A Note About Short Stature

These children are clearly shorter than their peers.
You will not need a growth curve to know they have short
stature. Short stature in the presence of adequate nutrition

and mental deficiency is a warning sign that the child suffers from a medical or genetic syndrome.

Normalized standards of growth have been obtained and are used by physicians and nurses to determine if a child is growing properly. The term "failure to thrive" is a medical term that means failure to gain weight at the appropriate rate. Short structure is the failure to grow in length at the appropriate rate.

If a child is undernourished (for any reason), the first result will be a failure to gain weight. Only after the malnutrition is longstanding will a failure to gain in length or stature begin. If the malnutrition begins after birth, the baby's birth length will be normal. In the disorders listed below, the children are usually born small and continue to grow poorly in height throughout life.

Any child who has mental dysfunction and one or more of the physical abnormalities listed above should have a genetic evaluation. Many individuals have these physical attributes without any mental dysfunction.

Chapter 12

Treatments for Children with Mental Dysfunction

There are many available treatments for children with mental handicaps, ranging from medicines to psychotherapy. This chapter describes the treatments available and indicates when each type of therapy is beneficial.

Megadose Vitamins

There is no such thing as a "smart pill." No medication has been shown to improve intelligence in all mentally handicapped children. If a child has a specific biochemical abnormality such as multiple carboxylase deficiency or homocystinuria (see Chapter 9), particular vitamin therapies can improve their mental function. *These megavitamin therapies only work for children who have these rare inborn errors of metabolism. Megavitamin therapy has no effect on children who do not have these rare disorders. By all means have your child evaluated by a geneticist for these problems, but if the evaluation is negative, do not subject your child to unnecessary and expensive vitamin treatments.*

Folic acid treatment has been suggested for the treatment of children with the Fragile X syndrome. There is, as yet, no scientific evidence to support any beneficial effect of high dose folic acid treatment of children with Fragile X syndrome. There are enough anecdotal reports (reports by doctors about individual patients, as opposed to large studies using many patients) of beneficial effects of folic acid to convince most doctors to try folic acid treatment in children with Fragile X syndrome, despite the lack of conclusive evidence (Fisch et al., 1988; Brown, 1989; Gustafson et al., 1985; Brown et al., 1986; Brown et al., 1984).

Parents of handicapped children are often desperate to find a pill or treatment to improve their child's mental functioning. Many travel great distances to doctors who claim to have miraculous results with various drug regimens. Beware of anyone who claims to have a treatment that works for all retarded or learning-disabled children. Check out anyone making these claims with your pediatrician or with the American Medical Association. Resist the temptation to try every new gimmick that comes on the market. Work with your doctors. If you read something about a miracle treatment, have your doctor check it out to see if there is any validity to it.

Hard work and appropriate therapy are what will optimize a handicap child's functioning, not pills.

Drugs

As mentioned in Chapter 4, stimulant medication such as Ritalin, Cylert, and Dexedrine can have dramatic beneficial effects for children with attention deficit disorders. These medicines can only be prescribed by a physician and require close physician follow-up to avoid side effects. If your child has attention deficit disorder, a trial of stimulant medication is recommended.

In some children, depression contributes to their dysfunction and antidepressant medication can be helpful. Like the stimulants, these medications are available only by prescription and children taking these medications require close medical supervision. Unlike the stimulants, antidepressant medications take several weeks to begin working, so give them at least six weeks before deciding that they are not helping your child.

Antipsychotic drugs such as Thorazine, Mellaril, Stelazine, Haldol and, rarely, lithium are used in children who are uncontrollable in classrooms and/or at home. These medications can sometimes take the edge off aggressive or hyperactive behavior in mentally handicapped children with behavior problems. These drugs can only be prescribed by a physician and children require close supervision while taking them.

Children with Tourette's syndrome can benefit tremendously from medication (Chapter 8). Stimulant medication can help the attention deficit disorder and Haldol can prevent the tics. Close medical supervision is required.

Other diseases listed in this book that cause mental dysfunction have their own treatments. It is most important to establish the diagnosis. This is accomplished by medical evaluations. Once the diagnosis is known, the appropriate therapies can be designed.

Diet

There is no specific dietary therapy that is beneficial to all children with mental dysfunction! As in vitamin therapy, specially designed diets can prevent mental retardation in children with specific diseases such as phenylketonuria, galactosemia, or hereditary fructose intolerance (see Chapter 10), so make sure that your child is evaluated for these diseases. If the evaluations are negative, however, resist the impulse to try all the fad diets continually appearing in the media.

I have never seen mental dysfunction caused by a food allergy. Many allergists claim to be able to improve mental performance in handicapped children by eliminated certain foods from the diet. As far as I am concerned, this is nonsense. Certainly food allergies exist, but the symptoms are diarrhea, vomiting, and failure to gain weight, not mental dysfunction. Not until malnutrition has progressed to starvation would these allergies impact on mental growth and development.

Please resist the temptation to try elaborate diets. Your efforts could be much better spent in participating in beneficial therapies for your child.

Eye Exercises

This topic was discussed in Chapter 4. Many optometrists claim to be able to treat learning disabilities with eye exercises. There is no evidence to show that these programs have any effect on a child's mental performance. The eye exercise programs can be extremely costly. The time and money spent in carrying out these useless programs could be much better spent in following beneficial programs for your child.

Infant Stimulation

Infant stimulation is the primary treatment for infants (children under two) with mental or physical handicaps. Infants may be identified because of a recognized disorder such as Down syndrome, or because of developmental delay.

A child without mental handicap will acquire normal developmental skills with no intervention. As long as the child receives parental affection and nutrition he will learn to roll over, sit up, walk, manipulate objects, and achieve the other developmental milestones without being taught. T. Berry Brazelton once described a child-rearing practice in an African tribe. The babies were worn in a backpack by their mother while she worked all day every day for the first 12 months of life. Even without ever having ever seen a Fischer-Price toy, Dr. Brazelton said, these children all acquired the appropriate developmental milestones on time!

Children with mental dysfunction do not acquire developmental skills without intervention. These children need to be *taught* skills other children learn on their own. This is what infant stimulation is all about. It is a combination of physical therapy, occupational therapy, and educational therapy, forming a comprehensive therapeutic program. It is certainly not just "playing with babies." Unfortunately, the term infant stimulation does not connote the seriousness or complexity of the therapies. There is absolutely no question that infant stimulation programs dramatically improve both the short-term and long-term prognosis for mentally handicapped children. Infant stimulation programs combined with medical interventions and Special Educational services have improved the ultimate prognosis for children with Down syndrome from near-certain institutionalization to semi-independent living and holding a job.

Usually parents are encouraged to participate in infant stimulation programs so the child can receive therapy on a continual basis.

Infant stimulation cannot do any harm to a child. If there is any question regarding the development of your infant, enroll him or her in an infant stimulation program as soon as possible. You can always discontinue the program if the problems are resolved.

Behavior Modification

Behavior modification is a technique based on the concept of *operant conditioning*. Operant conditioning involves changing a child's behavior by the systematic use of rewards and punishments. Conditioning was first demonstrated in the famous experiments now known as Pavlov's dogs. Pavlov was attempting to study the timing of salivary responses in dogs. He would place meat powder in the dogs' mouths and record how long it took for them to begin salivating. At first the dogs began to salivate after the powder was placed in their mouths. Later, however, the dogs began to salivate before the food was placed in their mouths, after just seeing the food. Eventually, the dogs began salivating as soon as the experimenter entered the room.

The dogs had "learned" to respond to the sight of the experimenter with salivation. This form of learning is called conditioning. The sight of the experimenter is called the stimulus and the salivation is called the response.

After Pavlov's description of conditioned responses, other scientists, including B. F. Skinner, began to experiment with the technique. What they discovered was that, with animals (and subsequently, people), by rewarding desirable behaviors and/or punishing undesirable behaviors, individuals could be trained to perform almost any behavior. In operant conditioning, use of rewards is called positive reinforcement and use of punishments is called negative reinforcement. Using the techniques of operant conditioning, scientists could train animals to perform incredible feats. The Ping-Pong-playing pigeons of B. F. Skinner and cats who use the toilet are two examples of the power of this technique.

Behavior modification uses the same techniques of operant conditioning with negative and/or positive reinforcements. All parents and teachers use rewards and/or punishments to some extent. Allowances are withheld for failure to do chores, presents are given for a good grade, etc. Behavior modification differs from these common interventions because it requires vigilance and consistency. Behavior modification techniques can be quite powerful in eliminating undesirable behaviors in children.

Behavior modification techniques are a form of training. As such they can be extremely successful in eliminating unwanted behaviors in children, but do not solve the problem causing the behavior. As an example, let us consider a six-year-old child who cries whenever his mother leaves the room. Behavior modification techniques would involve a negative reinforcement (punishment) every time the child cried when the mother left the room. At this age negative reinforcements are usually in the form of "time-outs." If a child exhibits undesirable behavior he or she will be given a "time-out." He will either be sent to a corner of the room or into a different room for a fixed period of time. "Time-outs" are extremely painful for children as it deprives of them of all human contact. Soon the child will learn that crying causes the "time-outs," and since the "time-outs" are unpleasant, the child will soon stop crying.

Although this form of behavior modification can be extremely effective in eliminating behaviors, the drawback is that nothing has been done about the cause of the problem.

Another way to approach the same child involves enlisting the aid of child psychiatrist, child psychologist, or social worker. Using specialized techniques developed for these situations, the therapist may be able to determine that the child's crying is due to separation anxiety relating to the death of a grandparent. Once the source of the problem is determined, therapy can be initiated to allow resolution of the problem *and* elimination of the undesirable behavior.

If behavior modification techniques were used with this child, the problem of the separation anxiety would remain. Often in these situations the children will "symptom-substitute" and have another symptom or problem, such as bedwetting or hitting. Then behavior modification could be used again to stop these behaviors, but new problems are likely to result. In any event, the true reason for the original undesirable behavior has remained unresolved.

Behavior modification is extremely popular because it gets results. Almost any behavior in any child can be eliminated with appropriate behavior modification techniques. However, the goal of parenting is not the creation of an individual with no undesirable behaviors. The goal of parenting is to produce a child with the fewest possible unresolved psychological and physical problems.

I believe behavior modification does have its place in the care of mentally handicapped children, but only after all other efforts to identify and treat the causes of the disruptive behavior have been exhausted. For autistic children, for example, behavior modification techniques are currently the only effective means of modeling behavior because the central problems are inaccessible to medical therapy or psychotherapy. Severely and profoundly retarded children are also resistant to almost all other forms of therapy except behavior modification.

Therefore, I believe behavior modification can be useful in controlling undesirable behaviors in children but should only be used sparingly, and only as a last resort.

When deciding whether or not it is time to try behavior modification treatment with your child, it is important to weigh the pros and cons of the situation. You must decide whether or not the behavior can be tolerated for awhile until the child resolves the problem causing it.

For example, the parents of an eight-year-old boy named Joseph came to me. Joseph has Tourette's syndrome. They were considering trying behavior modification because Joseph had recently begun to wet the bed. Every night he would have a urinary accident and his mother would have to give him a bath, change his clothes, and change the sheets and blankets. Their pediatrician had suggested that Joseph's parents let him lie in the wet sheets and refuse to bathe him, change him, or give him any attention. This is a form of behavior modification.

I asked the parents if Joseph's bed-wetting in its present form was intolerable. Their answer was yes. We then discussed why the accidents were occurring; they were probably a way of getting attention and comfort from his parents to alleviate his fears at nighttime. At my suggestion, we began a plan. I mediated, and Joseph and his parents developed a way to alleviate some of the anxieties he was feeling at night. We instituted a quiet time before bed when one of Joseph's parents would read to him or discuss the day's events. I also explained to Joseph that his accidents and the resulting work for his mother were taking too much of a toll. I suggested that he should wear a diaper at night, so if he had an accident he wouldn't need to have his pajamas and sheets changed, and he probably wouldn't even wake up. Joseph hated wearing the diapers, but agreed to do so in exchange for the quiet time with his parents. This plan worked well, and within two months the diapers were no longer necessary and the quiet times continued.

In this case I was able to modify the effect of Joseph's behavior so it could be tolerated by his parents for the period of time necessary to correct the fundamental problem (his nocturnal anxiety). It could also be noted that by putting him in a diaper it negated the gain of his behavior, namely the attention of his mother.

Sometimes, however, behaviors cannot be tolerated, and no other therapies (psychological or medical) have succeeded. In these cases behavior modification may be the only remedy for the situation. Just keep in mind that behavior modification treats the symptom, not the problem.

Educational Therapy

Academic tutoring is the cornerstone of educational therapy for educable retarded children (IQs 55–69) and children with learning disabilities. After appropriate testing determines a child's strengths and weaknesses, educational therapy will help to support the weaknesses and develop the strengths. This process is called remediation. Usually this occurs in a school setting in Special Education programs. Private tutors are available to work with your child at home and can be of tremendous benefit for your child. Unfortunately, insurance coverage rarely reimburses for educational services, despite their unquestioned value in obtaining the best results for handicapped children.

Alternative Educational Methods

Sometimes a child's disability is so complete in a given area that remediation is impossible. For example, some dyslexic children will never be able to learn to read. Continually trying to teach these children how to read is not only useless, but causes frustration and low self-esteem in the child. Unfortunately, remediation is what educators know how to do and it is what they usually offer. Often I see a learning-disabled high-school student in a "learning disabilities math class" where fractions are (unsuccessfully) taught. You, as parents, along with your physicians, may have to say, enough already; let's look for alternatives. Fortunately, in the modern world, there are alternative forms of acquiring and disseminating information other than by reading and writing. Dyslexic children can listen to books recorded for the blind. These tapes are available at no cost and any book can be obtained with sufficient advance notice by contacting blind service organizations (see the Appendix). Some children who have difficulty with handwriting and/or spelling can use word processors. Laptop portable computers make classroom word processing feasible. Tape recorders can be used to take notes or write compositions. Oral examinations can be given. There *are* alternatives. If your child is not progressing in his or her current program, alternative educational methods may be the answer. The impetus will almost certainly have to come from you, however. If the school district suggests alternative methods they would have to pay for the equipment.

Occupational and Physical Therapy

Many occupational and physical therapists specialize in treating handicapped children. These professionals will evaluate your child's physical strengths and weaknesses and design treatment programs to help the weaknesses. Fine motor and gross motor skills, strength, and daily living skills (handwriting, eating with utensils, etc.) can all be taught by these professionals.

As with infant stimulation, occupational and physical therapy can do no harm to children, and the benefits can be substantial. Therefore if there is any question that your child has physical problems, obtain a physical or occupational therapy evaluation as soon as possible. Unlike tu-

toring, many insurance companies will reimburse for phy-
sician-ordered OT and PT. The therapists will also demonstrate exercises and games that you can perform with
your child on your own.

Speech Therapy

Speech therapists specialize in the diagnosis and treatment of children and adults with speech problems. Since
delayed speech is one of the most frequent initial problems
observed in handicapped children, speech therapists are in
the forefront of the care of handicapped children. Speech
therapists provide essential services for handicapped children that cannot be duplicated by other professionals.

Many insurance carriers will reimburse for speech
therapy and most special education districts employ speech
therapists for their students. I urge you to seek speech
therapy for your child if he or she has any difficulties in
speech, including inappropriate inflection, echoing what
other people say, too few words in his spoken or receptive
vocabulary, or inappropriate language in social situations.
(See Chapter 13 for further discussion.)

Psychotherapy

Psychotherapy is a valuable part of the total treatment
of mentally handicapped children. Most mentally handicapped children will benefit from psychological therapy.
Many professionals are capable of performing psychotherapy with children. Pediatric social workers, child psychologists, and child psychiatrists are trained professionals. For

young children, techniques of play therapy and art therapy can have dramatic results in resolving psychological problems.

Choosing the proper therapist for your child is important. It is vital that your child be comfortable with the therapist you have chosen. The most famous child psychiatrist in the world will do your child no good if he or she is unable to engage your child. Feel free to ask for a referral to another therapist if you think that your child is not benefiting from the therapist you have chosen. Perhaps your child will relate better to a man than a woman, or vice versa. It is important that the child and therapist establish a good relationship.

The total care of a handicapped child will involve various combinations of the therapies discussed in this chapter. It is important to use your doctor as a guide to services that can benefit your child. Remember to have your child's treatment program reevaluated periodically to assess if changes are needed. You do not want to force a round peg into a square hole.

Chapter 13

What Should I Do for My Mentally Handicapped Child?

This chapter provides information and advice about how to proceed when you believe your child may have a mental handicap. Caring for a child with a mental or physical handicap becomes a lifelong vocation. The experience can be devastating, but with adequate information and support, you can provide the necessary service for your handicapped child without destroying your family life. You will need to learn to create a balance to allow for sufficient time with your spouse and other children. This chapter outlines how to obtain the necessary medical and therapeutic services for your child, and discusses strategies to help you keep your family together and thriving.

Many parents take their child to many doctors in many different cities in an attempt to find someone who can help. This is an exhausting, expensive, and usually unnecessary process. This chapter describes a reasonable approach to obtaining a diagnosis and treatment for a mentally handicapped child.

It is vital for your child's sake, as well as your own peace of mind, that all possible medical conditions have been evaluated, and that your child is reevaluated annually. Your child's problem may finally be understood next week, next month, or next year, so it is important to keep in contact with the specialists on a yearly basis so that they can determine if there is any new diagnosis or treatment for your child.

The First Step

As soon as you become concerned that your child may have a mental handicap, the first step is to notify your child's primary physician, the child's "doctor." He or she will usually be a pediatrician, family practitioner, or general practitioner. All children should have a primary physician.

The initial concern regarding a possible mental handicap in your child may come from you, your spouse, or other family member, a physician's observation, or from a day-care center or school. Table 12 lists possible first indications of mental handicap in infants and children.

Each problem requires a different intervention and evaluation.

Vision

Infants who are blind or severely visually handicapped at birth will not be able to focus on faces or follow objects

Table 12. Indications of Handicaps in Infants and Children

Problem
Physical Handicap
    Vision
    Hearing
    Coordination
    Fine motor
    Gross motor
Mental Handicap
    Developmental delay
    Delayed speech
    Mental retardation
    Learning disability
    Loss of milestones
Emotional Handicap
    Aggressive behavior
    Self-mutilation
    Self-stimulatory behavior (rocking,
        head-banging, etc.)

visually. However, many newborns with normal eyesight
will not be able to perform these functions for several
weeks. Such children may also have unusual jerking eye
movements called nystagmus. If your child is not focusing
on your face or following your movements by six weeks
of age, take the baby to see a pediatric ophthalmologist
(an eye doctor who specializes in children). The doctor
will examine the baby and perform a test known as an
ERG (electroretinogram) to see if the proper electrical signals are sent from the eyes to the brain after lights are
flashed.

Children who are not blind but have poor vision are
more difficult to diagnose. The first indication that a child

may have vision problems may be the observation that the child sits extremely close to the television set or holds his head very close to the pages of a book. One parent told me that she was continually wiping nose prints off her television screen and, when her daughter drew pictures, her cheek often touched the paper. Abnormal jerking eye movements may alert you or your doctor to vision problems in an infant or toddler.

Once your child enters school, vision is screened routinely. You may receive a notice from the school nurse to have your child's vision examined. If you are concerned about a child's vision, you must see an ophthalmologist (not an optometrist), and preferably an ophthalmologist who specializes in children (pediatric ophthalmologist). In contrast to optometrists, ophthalmologists are doctors and surgeons who can complete a medical and, if necessary, surgical evaluation of your child's eyes and vision.

If your child has mild nearsightedness (myopia) or a simple "lazy eye" (amblyopia) and no other problems, a visit to the ophthalmologist is all you need to do. On the other hand, if your child is blind, has dislocated lenses (ectopia lentis), severe nearsightedness (severe myopia), corneal cloudiness, cataract, defect of the iris (colored portion of the eye) or retina (back of the eye) (coloboma), glaucoma, and/or other mental or physical problems, a genetic evaluation is advisable.

Hearing

If an infant is deaf, it is extremely important to recognize this as soon as possible, because proper visual and touching stimulation can be substituted for aural stimulation. Failure to recognize deafness in infancy and to institute appropriate therapy can result in severe emotional problems for the child, including the devastating illness known as autism.

It is difficult to determine if an infant is deaf by simple observation. This is because an infant will respond to movements and faces in addition to sound. Even if you stand behind a child and clap your hands, the child may feel the air move or see the movement of your hands.

One clue that your child may have a hearing problem is the structure of his ears. Abnormally shaped earlobes, or earlobes that are tilted forward or backwards, or extra pieces of skin (called skin tags) near one or both ears are all warning signs that your child may have a hearing problem. He should be taken to an ear, nose, and throat specialist (ENT) as soon as possible.

If you are concerned about your infant or child's hearing, a special battery of tests can be performed by the ENT doctor to evaluate his hearing. The ENT doctor will perform a physical examination to determine if the ear structure is normal. A tympanogram will determine if the eardrum is moving properly and an audio-evoked response will determine if the proper electrical signals are being sent to the brain when sounds are played.

Children who are not deaf at birth can still develop progressive hearing loss as they grow older. Such children may hear reasonably well in infancy, only to have their hearing deteriorate as they grow. Recurrent problems with ear infections and fluid accumulation behind the ear (serous otitis media) can also affect hearing. The first sign that a child may have a hearing loss may be a delay in developing speech, or development of indistinct speech patterns.

Once a child enters school, hearing tests (called audiometry) are performed routinely. You should be informed of any problems by the school nurse. If any hearing problems are noted, an evaluation by an ENT specialist is necessary as soon as possible.

If a problem with hearing is present in your child, a genetic evaluation is necessary. Many genetic diseases can cause hearing loss, and it will important to establish if your child has one of these problems for all the reasons outlined in the first chapter.

Coordination, Fine Motor Skills, and Gross Motor Skills

Difficulties with coordination are not usually obvious to parents until the second year of life, when children begin to walk, drink from a cup, ride a tricycle, color with crayons, and hold eating utensils. Sometimes a child will fall down frequently or be unable to manipulate a crayon. Sometimes these difficulties simply represent a delay in maturation. Some children develop motor skills at faster rates than other children even though they will eventually acquire these skills. If you are concerned that your child may have a coordination problem, consult your child's primary physician.

If the physician agrees that there is a possible problem, a referral to a pediatric neurologist (a doctor who specializes in the nervous system of children) should be made. The specialist can determine if there is a problem and if any special testing is required.

Mental Handicap: Developmental Delay

Deciding whether or not a child has true developmental delay is one of the most difficult judgments a primary physician has to make. Because different children develop different skills at varying ages, it is often difficult to decide whether a child who is slow to develop a skill has a problem or is just a "late bloomer." For example, some perfectly normal children *never* crawl. Some scoot or roll as a means of locomotion and begin walking on schedule.

I often see parents with handicapped children who tell me, "I kept telling my pediatrician that something was wrong and he kept telling me that everything was OK," or "From the moment he was born I knew something was wrong, but no one, especially my doctors, would believe me."

In this situation, the parents are blaming their pediatricians for not accepting their concerns regarding the development of their child. One must put the situation into perspective, however. It is very common for parents to be concerned about the development of their children, myself included. My first child, Rachel, walked when she was a year old. She had a friend who began to walk at nine months of age. I knew that "normal" children can begin to walk as late as 15 months, so I was not overly concerned. My second child, Sam, did not begin walking until 14 months of age. Even though I *knew* that this was still within the normal range of child development, I *was* concerned. Our pediatrician was reassuring, of course, because everything else was progressing well. Sam did begin to walk and is now a "normal" second-grader.

The point is, if Sam did not begin to walk at 14 months, and was still not walking at 18 months, our pediatrician would not have been wrong in his attempts to reassure us at the 14-month checkup. The overwhelming majority of parents who have concerns regarding their child's development who are reassured by their pediatrician that their child is healthy actually do have "normal" children who are developing at slightly different rates than their peers or siblings.

If your primary physician agrees with your concerns regarding your child's development, or if he or she notices a delay, then it is time to have a complete developmental evaluation. Another reason for a complete developmental evaluation is if you feel that your concerns regarding developmental delay in your child are real, and are not being addressed by your primary physician.

Developmental evaluations are performed by various professionals. You may have to do some research to find out who is competent to perform this testing in your location. A relatively new subspeciality in pediatrics is developmental pediatrics. These specialists are trained in the evaluation and treatment of children with developmental delay and other mental handicaps, in addition to their pediatric training. A developmental pediatrician is qualified to perform a developmental assessment. A pediatric neurologist, a neurologist who specializes in the problems of children, will be able to perform the evaluation or to refer you to a clinical psychologist, physical therapist, or occupational therapist qualified to perform developmental evaluations.

The developmental evaluation examines your child's accomplishments using specific tests (called instruments) of infant development. The two most popular tests are called the Bayley Test of Infant Development and the Denver Developmental Test. The results of this testing can be difficult for a layperson to interpret or understand. It is important for you to meet with the examiner and keep asking questions until you are satisfied that you understand the conclusions of the testing. Although it may be reassuring to hear that "We don't think there is anything to worry about," be sure to ask specific questions regarding your concerns, such as, "Does the testing show that there is a problem in any area for my child?" "Are the results completely normal?"

If the testing is abnormal, you will embark upon the next series of evaluations. A neurological assessment by a pediatric neurologist and a genetic evaluation are necessary at this time. The neurologist can assess if there are any problems such as epilepsy, abnormal brain structure, or muscle problems in your baby. The geneticist will determine if your baby is suffering from a genetic disease, biochemical problem, or birth defect syndrome.

Children who are identified as having developmental delay need physical and occupational therapy. For infants these programs are called infant stimulation. This type of therapy helps children build up the physical skills required to master the tasks of development and are quite valuable for children with developmental delay from any cause. One way to think about it is that "normal" children develop the necessary skills with minimal help, but handicapped children will need to be taught these skills.

As a child with developmental delay grows, new information may become available to allow more accurate assessments of his or her mental capabilities. Parents and physicians must be alert to any new problems developing in the child and begin treatment promptly. It is particularly important to make sure that hearing and vision are checked thoroughly at regular intervals.

Delayed Speech

Another way children with mental handicaps can be identified is through delayed development of speech. Most children will begin to say ma-ma and da-da with specific reference to their parents by 18 months of age. By two years old they should have a vocabulary of at least 50 words. By age three they should be saying sentences containing at least three words. Children should understand and be able to follow simple commands by 18 months of age, and more complex commands by two years of age.

Somewhere in the period between 18 months and two years, if a child is not developing any language abilities, a speech evaluation should be performed. This will involve an evaluation of hearing by an ear, nose, and throat specialist (ENT) and evaluation by a speech therapist. Children who are hard of hearing do not develop speech at normal rates. Children whose delayed speech is caused by hearing problems are usually also delayed in understanding speech.

Other children may have poor tongue or palate movements, causing speech delay. Children with these problems usually understand speech normally.

The most common outcome of the hearing and speech evaluations, however, is that no explanation can be found for the delayed speech.

If the speech evaluations confirm that the child has

a speech problem, speech therapy should begin immediately. In addition, a complete genetic and neurologic evaluation is also advised as soon as the diagnosis of a speech problem is made. This is because intellectual dysfunction is the most common cause of delayed speech. Any child who is diagnosed as having intellectual dysfunction deserves a complete evaluation to establish a diagnosis and to determine if the child has a medically treatable form of mental dysfunction.

Mental Retardation

As discussed in Chapter 1, mental retardation is defined in terms of scores on intelligence tests in combination with an evaluation of the child's social, emotional, and adaptive skills. In infancy, intelligence testing involves mainly assessing the development of motor skills. After two years of age reliable measurements of intellectual capabilities can be obtained. Mentally retarded children often (but not always) have developmental delay in infancy and delayed speech during toddlerhood. Mentally retarded children also need a complete genetic and neurological evaluation. The cause of mental retardation can be established for approximately half of all severely retarded children (see Introduction). The causes may be genetic, a multiple malformation syndrome or other birth defect, or prenatal or postnatal injury.

The treatment for children with mental retardation is based on each individual child's particular strengths and weaknesses. Most preschool children will require both physical therapy to help them learn physical skills and educational therapy (tutoring) to help them master intellectual skills. The earlier this intervention begins, the better the eventual outcome will be. For example, early intervention and continued therapy has drastically altered the prognosis of children with Down syndrome (see Chapter 6).

Learning Disability

As discussed in Chapter 4, children with learning disabilities have normal IQs but are unable to progress normally in school for various reasons. This category includes children with hyperactivity (attention deficit disorder). As soon as a child is suspected to have a learning disability, testing should be performed as soon as possible. If testing confirms a disability, a neurologic and genetic evaluation is necessary. If there is an emotional component to the problem, psychiatric or psychological evaluation and treatment are also needed.

Learning disabilities testing defines the problem areas of each child so appropriate tutoring programs can be designed. Sometimes alternative learning methods, such as oral examinations, or the use of word processors, can be extremely helpful. It is important to involve your doctor (see below) in school decisions and in formulating private tutoring plans so that appropriate treatment plans can be designed. It is also important to periodically review the treatment plan with teachers, other school staff, and any private tutors, to see if the therapeutic program is effective. It is vital for parents to be involved with the decisions regarding school placement and treatment plans. No one knows as much about a child as his parents. A detailed section discussing school placements follows later in this chapter.

Loss of Milestones

The definition and diagnosis of loss of milestones was discussed in detail in Chapter 7. As soon as a child is suspected to have a loss of milestones, an immediate evaluation by a pediatric neurologist is needed to make sure that a brain tumor or other treatable problem is not present. The neurologist's evaluation may include X rays of the brain (CT scans and MRI scans) and electrical tests of the muscles and nerves called Electromylography (EMG) and Nerve Conduction Studies, respectively. The electrical studies may suggest a genetic disease such as a lysosomal storage disease (see Chapter 9). If the neurologist is unable to establish the cause of the loss of milestones, a biochemical genetic evaluation is needed.

Emotional Handicaps

Autism is a severe mental disturbance in children. Autistic children, from early infancy, do not respond to other people, including their parents. As they grow older they usually engage in self-stimulatory behavior such as incessant rocking or head-banging. There is no proven medical cause for autism although many theories exist. Most scientists think autism involves some kind of chemical imbalance or defective brain structure.

Although some treatment plans have had some limited success with some autistic children, most autistic chil-

dren eventually require institutionalization. All children diagnosed as being autistic or having autistic-like symptoms
should have their hearing checked and have a genetic evaluation. This is because deaf children can become autistic
and because there are three diseases (Fragile X syndrome,
Rett's syndrome, and Cornelia de Lange syndrome) whose
symptoms can mimic autism (Chapter 8).

Self-mutilation and physical aggression are two other
severe problems that can have a genetic basis (Chapter 8).

Milder forms of emotional disturbance may be apparent in interactions with other children, brothers and
sisters, or teachers. Children with learning disabilities often
develop behavioral problems or emotional disturbances.

Symptoms of depression in children are quite variable.
Some children sleep a lot, others complain of headaches
or stomachaches that have no demonstrable physical basis.

A child who has behavior problems, emotional problems, or repeated physical complaints with no discovered
physical basis needs to have a psychiatric or psychological
evaluation. If, however, the child is also having academic
problems in school, a learning disabilities evaluation is also
important. Teachers commonly complain about children
who have undiagnosed learning disabilities: "If he would
only try harder, I know he could do the work," or "He's
always daydreaming and looking out the window," or
"He's just lazy." These statements should alert you as a
parent to the possibility of a learning disability, and your
child should be evaluated as soon as possible (see Chapter
4). If a learning disability is present, proceed to the genetic
and neurological evaluations, as described in previous sections.

The treatments for children with emotional disorders
vary with the diagnosed cause of the problem. Counseling

by a psychiatrist, psychologist, or social worker is an important part of the treatment, regardless of the cause of the problem. Many parents have difficulty admitting that their child may need this kind of help. Do not allow your feelings (anger, embarrassment, self-consciousness) to interfere with obtaining therapy for your child. Psychotherapy can literally save your child's life. If your child's therapist suggests family therapy, when the entire family participates in the therapeutic process, you owe it to your child to participate. For emotionally handicapped children, psychotherapy is as important as eyeglasses are for a nearsighted child. Without therapy the child can flounder and fail in school, and with therapy, the child can succeed.

Once you have established that your child has a mental handicap, the next steps are to choose a doctor and to develop a treatment plan. The remainder of this chapter discusses these two issues. Before proceeding to this subject, I want to stress an important aspect of routine pediatric care that needs modification for children with potential mental handicap.

DPT Immunizations

Routine care for infants involves immunizations against diphtheria, pertussis, and tetanus. This is accomplished by administering a series of shots with a vaccine (DPT shots). Usually a DPT shot is given at two months of age, four months of age, and six months of age, followed by "booster" shots at 18 months, and before entering kindergarten. In most states, proof of immunizations is required before a child can be enrolled in public school.

Children with a neurological handicap can have bad reactions to the pertussis component of the DPT vaccine. The reaction can cause seizures and permanent brain injury. If there is any question regarding a child being neurologically handicapped, he should not receive a DPT immunization. Make sure that your doctor administers a *DT* vaccination. This contains the diphtheria and typhoid vaccines without the pertussis vaccine. There are new pertussis vaccines that may be safe for neurologically handicapped children, but for now *no child suspected of having neurological dysfunction should receive a DPT vaccination.*

Although there have been claims that "normal" children have been permanently damaged by the pertussis vaccine, this has not been proven. Pertussis (whooping cough) is an extremely serious illness in infancy that results in months of illness, and can even be fatal. So, if your child is not neurologically handicapped, he or she should receive the usual DPT vaccination.

Choosing a Doctor

It is important to choose one physician to be primarily responsible for coordinating the care and treatment of your child. There will be two aspects to your child's care, so-called primary care pediatrics provided to all children, and specialized care for the particular needs of your handicapped child.

Following the initial developing, genetic, and neurological evaluations, there may be at least three physicians already involved in your child's care; the primary physician, the pediatric neurologist, and the geneticist. At this point, a specific division of labor should be established. It is important that everyone involved understand the exact role of each doctor. Confusion must be avoided at all costs. Confusion can lead to ruffled feathers and bruised egos, but more importantly it can lead to important treatment issues "slipping through the cracks." You do not want to hear, "I thought Dr. Johnson was doing hearing tests every six months," when your three-year-old has never had a hearing test.

To avoid this, you can divide medical responsibilities between the primary physician and one specialist. Your pediatrician can be given responsibility for primary care issues such as ear infections and immunizations, while the specialist can coordinate the special care indicated by your child's problems. This is the most common arrangement, and usually works well if the two physicians involved have a good working relationship. You must inform your primary physician of your plan to divide the responsibilities in this manner. You must ask both physicians involved if they have any problem with this arrangement. There may be a personality conflict between the two of them, making it impossible for them to work well together. Your primary physician may tell you that he or she is perfectly able to handle your child's problem and would resent interference from the specialist.

If one or both of the physicians involved are not comfortable with the arrangement you have chosen, you will have to make another decision. You can change one or both physicians, or decide to agree to an alternate arrangement. It is important to realize that the ultimate decision is *yours*, and that this decision is one of the single most important decisions you will make during the life of your child. Don't hesitate to get a second opinion, or to interview various primary physicians and specialists. You must establish relationships with physicians with whom you are comfortable, because care of a handicapped child is a lifelong partnership. Consider competence, experience, accessibility, and personality in making your decision. If feelings are hurt, so be it. Your highest priority and most important responsibility is to select the physicians you feel are best for you and your child. Don't allow yourself to be forced into a position you are not comfortable with.

The obvious choice for the primary coordinator is your primary physician. He or she can act as a mediator between you and the specialists. Even if your child has a condition requiring a specialist's care, for example, a seizure disorder (epilepsy), your primary physician can still be the primary coordinator for all his care. The advantage of using your primary physician for general health care for your child is that he or she is more accessible, used to handling telephone enquiries from patients, and is willing and able to handle general pediatric care issues. Regardless of your baby's special problems, he or she can have ear infections, cuts and falls, and will still need immunizations and checkups.

Although an individual specialist may have more experience with your child's particular problems, he or she may be hard to reach on a Sunday night if your baby has a high fever. Many primary physicians are willing and anxious to participate actively in serving the special needs of handicapped children. I personally welcome such involvement. In these cases, I communicate directly with the primary physician and inform him or her of the special monitoring, precautions, and treatments needed for the child's disorder. For example, if a child has Down syndrome and the parents decide to split care between myself and a general pediatrician, I would make sure that hearing tests are performed, and that routine orthopedic (bone) and dental visits are made and that the child receives physical therapy, infant stimulation, occupational therapy, and tutoring. The general pediatrician would take care of primary-care needs, such as immunizations, school physicals, and routine checkups.

If the parents decided to place total responsibility in the hands of the general pediatrician, I would communicate the special needs of the child to the pediatrician, and he or she would take responsibility for assuring that the necessary interventions were obtained. As a specialist, I would still see the child intermittently in my office because I have more experience working with Down syndrome children and may be able recognize developing problems earlier than a general pediatrician; but all the other care for this child could be coordinated through the pediatrician. This arrangement usually works quite well.

You should always have a primary physician involved in the care of your child. Specialists can often overlook basic-care issues such as immunizations, and a visit to a specialist for a school physical is probably more time-consuming and expensive than a visit to a general pediatrician's office. In addition, your pediatrician will probably have more experience (and interest) in handling issues such as fevers, rashes, and toilet training than a specialist.

An alternative to a single specialist's individual care is a hospital-based specialty clinic staffed by several doctors with different specialities devoted to caring for children with particular problems. These clinics are usually associated with large teaching hospitals and are called multidisciplinary clinics. For example, a clinic for cranio-facial anomalies (abnormal structures in the face, skull, and mouth) may be staffed by geneticists, plastic surgeons, oral surgeons, dentists, speech therapists, and nutritionists. In a single visit (and usually a single charge), children can be evaluated by all these specialists and the "entire team" will recommend a treatment plan.

The advantage of these multidisciplinary clinics is obvious. You can take care of most of your child's special needs with one visit, rather than several individual visits to different specialists. The cost for the single clinic visit is usually less than the individual office visits. The disadvantage to such clinics is that because of their design, they are more impersonal than a private physician. This is because the clinic staff available in a given month changes. You may see one plastic surgeon in June, a second in July, and a third in August. It is up to you whether you feel comfortable in a clinic arrangement or prefer a private setting. It is important to realize that you may be able to get exactly the same quality of care from a network of individual experienced specialists as from a multidisciplinary clinic.

For some rare diseases such as tuberous sclerosis, or neurofibromatosis (see Appendix), clinics may only exist in a few places in the country. You may wish to travel and take your child to such a clinic once, or periodically, to make sure that he or she is receiving optimum care.

In any event, it is essential to *decide* which doctors or clinics will have primary responsibility for particular aspects of your child's care. You must also notify the physicians involved of your decision and make sure that they are *comfortable* with the arrangement. Only after this has been accomplished can you get down to business, the care and treatment of your handicapped child.

Developing a Treatment Plan

A treatment plan must be tailored to each individual child. It is important to involve people with experience in caring for and treating mentally handicapped children. Here again, your choice of a doctor to care for your child is important. The coordinator of your child's special needs will make sure that appropriate testing is performed and will suggest who should be involved in the care of your child, and what they should be doing.

Prior to school age, you and your doctors will be on your own regarding school placements. Most communities have preschool facilities with special classes or services for handicapped children. Many hospitals and schools have parent-infant programs to help parents help their children. It is up to you and your doctor to find an acceptable placement or to obtain the necessary services at home. Whatever you decide, it will be important to periodically reevaluate whatever treatment plan is used to make sure that it is helping your child. If the child is in a preschool, this reevaluation will include a school *staffing*, a meeting of all the individuals involved in your child's care to discuss your child's progress and ideas for future treatments or placements. Participants in the staffing can include you and your child's doctor, teachers, school nurses, therapists, psychologists, etc.

If your child is of school age, you need to decide whether to place your child in a private facility or to enter

the public school system. Most people decide to give the
public school system a try. The following section contains
advice on dealing with public school systems.

Dealing with the School Districts

In the United States, school districts are *mandated*
by federal law to provide your child with an appropriate
education (see Chapter 14). If the school district cannot
provide necessary services, they must pay for the child to
attend a private facility that can provide the necessary treatment. This is your right, and you must not be intimidated.
Sometimes parents have had to hire lawyers and sue school
districts to force them to provide necessary services for a
child.

Children with no identified problems enter kindergarten without fanfare or testing. If a child has already
been identified as having a problem, the school district
will decide on the appropriate placement and treatments
for your child. This decision involves reviewing your
child's records and the results of previous testing, discus-
sions with you, and probably their own evaluation of your
child. Following their evaluation, they will meet with you
(and, hopefully, your doctor) to inform you of their decision regarding placement and treatment.

If you and/or your doctor do not agree with their
placement, you can try to plead your case at that time.
In my experience, however, is better to give the school
district's placement a try. It is important not to force the
school district into placing your child in a regular (mainstream) classroom because of your fears that your child
will be stigmatized in a special placement. Floundering in

a mainstream classroom will do more harm to your child's self-image than the stigma of being in a "special ed" classroom. If your doctor and the school district agree that an alternate placement is advisable, please give it a try, for your child's sake.

Many school districts have adequate Special Education facilities and can provide the necessary treatment for handicapped children. However, with dwindling funding for these facilities, any given school district may not be able to provide the necessary services for any given child. Use your doctor as a guide and as a teammate to decide if your child is getting the proper services. Sometimes parents have to fight for this right for their children.

On the other hand, it is important to remember that the school districts want exactly the same thing for your child that you do, namely the best possible education. They have experience dealing with mentally handicapped children and therefore their suggestions for therapy and placements should be given a chance. A good rule of thumb is not to reject a placement before you have tried it. Unless you have an urgent reason to object to a suggested placement it is a good idea to follow the initial recommendations of the school district.

However, if after several months you believe that the placement is not helping your child, then it is time to request a staffing to discuss your concerns regarding the current placement. Ask your doctor to attend.

It is unwise to develop an adversarial relationship with the school district. Unless it is unavoidable, friendly relations work best. It is very helpful to involve your doctor. He or she will be acting solely for the benefit of your child. Financial issues, classroom size, and student-teacher ratios will not enter into your doctor's judgment. He or she will also be able to give the school district an independent evaluation and therapeutic suggestions for your child.

Enrolling your child in a private school gives you more control over his or her educational destiny than a public school placement. However, private schools can be extremely expensive and may not provide services superior to the public school special education district. The decision is yours alone to make. Use your doctor as an advisor and aide in making these decisions.

Many parents with handicapped children feel isolated. You need not go through this difficult process alone. Use your doctor as physician, advisor, ally, partner, and friend. Call your doctor frequently and share your experiences and your concerns. Invite your doctor to school staffings. You need not be alone. We are here to help you—use us.

I strongly urge parents to utilize support groups and service organization established for parents of children with mental handicaps. The Appendix contains a list of national organizations that provide services and support for handicapped individuals.

Reevaluation

It is important to have your child reevaluated by a specialist periodically. This is because research is continually providing new information about the causes and treatments of mental handicaps in children. I like to see children once a year so that I can observe their growth and development, evaluate their progress, and determine if anything new was discovered in the last year that could benefit the child.

Take Care of Yourself

Caring for any child is a challenge. Caring for a handicapped child is exhausting. You will spend hours driving to doctors' appointments, X-ray facilities, therapy sessions, and workshops. Many parents of handicapped children feel isolated. They see their friends, neighbors, and family members with their "normal" children and they feel that they are the only ones with handicapped children. They may want to hide their child to avoid stares or questions.

Let me assure you, if you have a handicapped child you are not alone. Three out of every hundred children have a birth defect and about the same number will be unable to progress in school. It is vital that you take advantages of services available to you. Two of the most frequent problems encountered by parents of handicapped children are burnout and marital problems. Since it may be difficult to find day-care or baby-sitting services for handicapped children, some parents literally never have any time away from their child. They are constantly "on call" for their child's needs. Having no time that is completely their own wears down parents to the point where they are no longer able to tolerate the constant demands on their time and energy. It is important for parents to find ways to free themselves each week for a few hours. This is usually accomplished by a daytime placement for the child. Another important resource to avoid burnout is a service known as respite care. Respite-care facilities are live-in facilities with professional staff who are trained to care for handicapped children. Most respite centers will take children for a period of one to two weeks. This is a necessary service so that the parents can unwind and recharge their batteries. Some parents feel guilty about utilizing respite-care facilities. They feel that they should be able to care for their children without any outside help. This attitude is wrong. It will do your child no good to have you burn out or sacrifice your marriage because you have run out of energy. Utilize the services that are available. Respite care can be as important for your child as it is to you.

Any family with a handicapped child is at high risk for divorce. Some statistics quote divorce rates as high as 80% for couples who have a handicapped child. Even in families who are able to stay together, problems can arise, like resentment by brothers and sisters for all the effort and attention lavished upon the handicapped child. My recommendation is to utilize available counseling services. Try individual psychotherapy, pastoral counseling, support groups, or any other services available to you and your spouse, and the siblings of a handicapped child. You need not feel guilty about having needs of your own that you want fulfilled by your spouse and your marriage. It is important to talk about these issues with your spouse.

Use all the resources available to you. You are not alone. Let us (the professional community) help you. Look at the Appendix. It contains a listing of national organizations that provide services for various disorders. All the founders and members of these many organizations have experienced the problems and challenges of raising a handicapped child. Not only can they help guide you in your efforts to obtain treatment for your child, they have "been there" and will understand.

Chapter 14

School Programs, Federal Laws, and Your Rights

Landmark legislation was passed by the federal government in 1975 that guarantees the right of *all* children to receive an appropriate education regardless of handicaps or disabilities. The law, P.L. 94-142, required that public schools must provide handicapped children from ages 3–21 with free and appropriate education including related services, with "due process" protections for parents. For children younger than three years and over 21, parents were on their own until 1988, when a new law, Federal Law 94-457, mandated that services be provided to children beginning at birth. States were given four years to comply with this new law (Meyen, 1982; Wright, 1982).

The law also gives "empowerment" to parents, which means you have the right to approve or disapprove of all educational plans for your child. Because these services are mandated by federal law they must be provided without cost to you.

The law also mandates that a handicapped child's special medical services, psychological services, and social services be provided.

It is up to each state to decide which agency or agencies are responsible for providing these services. Usually the educational system has primary responsibility for providing the educational services, but health departments may also become involved because of medical issues.

Under the new law, each state must provide programs for handicapped children of all ages. Since services for handicapped children under the age of three years were not mandated previously, programs for children from birth to three are usually separate from the programs for older children.

Programs to provide therapy and services for children from birth to three years are called Parent-Infant Programs or 0-3 Programs. These names are synonymous. These programs teach parents how to help their children at home, in addition to providing therapy at the centers. The amount of time each child will spend attending a Parent-Infant program will vary according to the severity of his problem and the resources of the facility. In any event, as is indicated by the name Parent-Infant Programs, parental participation is vital to the success of these programs for your child.

After the age of three years, if a child still requires special services, he or she will usually enter the auspices of the Special Education District in the area.

Included in special educational services are social services and psychological services.

Who Is Eligible for Special Services?

In order to be eligible for special services, testing must be performed to demonstrate the need for special services. Usually the school district or health department will want their own consultants to perform the evaluations but sometimes test results from professionals in the area are acceptable. The testing by the school district or health department should be provided free of charge.

Parent-Infant Programs usually require a developmental evaluation using the Bayley test or the Denver Developmental Test (see Chapter 2) prior to entrance into the program. The result of this test is reported in age equivalence. For example, parents of a 14-month-old child may be informed that he is functioning at a 9-month-old level. The results are divided into four skill types: gross motor skills, fine motor skills, language skills, and social-personal skills.

In order to qualify for special services (Parent-Infant Programs and 0–3 Programs), a child must be functioning at less than 70% age equivalence in one of the four areas or less than 75% age equivalence in two or more of the areas. For example, a 10-month-old infant would qualify for services if he or she was functioning at less than a 7-month level in any one of the four areas: gross motor, fine motor, language, or social-personal. If the child was functioning at a 7½-month level in one skill, but at more than that in the other 3, he or she would not qualify for services. However, functioning at the 7½-month level in any two of the areas would qualify the child for entry into Parent-Infant programs.

This situation reemphasizes the need to test your child

if you have any questions regarding his or her development. Do not be afraid that entry into such a program
will stigmatize your child. One of the goals of special programs is for the children to "graduate" from Parent-Infant
Programs and special education programs into mainstream
environments. Given the proper support and treatment for
various periods of time, many children are able to be successful in mainstream situations.

How Do I Get Services for My Child?

Since the federal law mandating services to children
ages 0–3 is new, it is not clear how referrals to programs
will be accomplished. My suggestion is to call your school
district and request information about referral to a Parent-Infant or 0–3 Program. For older children, referrals
usually come from classroom teachers who have noticed
a problem in a child, or at the suggestion of physicians
who are concerned about a physical or mental handicap.
Once the referrals are made, a series of evaluations will
usually be performed. Psychological, educational, and social assessments of your child will be made at this time.

After the evaluations are completed, you will meet
with all of the individuals who performed the various evaluations, a representative of the school district, and your
child's teachers. Although different school districts have
different names for this meeting, the most common term
is a *placement* staffing. Whatever the meeting is called, its
purpose is to inform you of your child's test results, the
conclusions of the school district, and the placement recommendation, or *individual educational plan* (abbreviated
IEP) suggested by the school district. This meeting is

mandated by law. A record of this meeting is kept (called minutes) and you will be asked to sign a paper indicating your attendance. At the conclusion of the meeting you may be asked to sign a document indicating your agreement with the suggested placement. Do not sign this document unless and until you are satisfied that this placement is the one that will most benefit your child!

This meeting will discuss the results of all the tests and evaluations, and a recommendation for placement or programs will be made. These meetings can be extremely difficult for parents to handle. You will be confronted by a tremendous amount of information, often in unfamiliar terminology. You may become sad, emotionally distraught, or angry because of some of the things you may hear. This will make understanding and interpreting the conclusions of this meeting even more difficult for you. For all these reasons, I have four firm recommendations regarding parents' attendance at school meetings.

1. *Both parents* should attend, or a second supportive friend or relative if one spouse cannot attend. This will give you emotional support and allow both of you to make an informed decision that will have an enormous impact on your child's life.

2. Ask a professional familiar with your child and with staffings to accompany you to the meeting. The professional will be able to understand all the terminology and interpret the findings for you. In addition, the professional will be able to explain the placements discussed in the meeting.

3. When you don't understand something, ask a question. Do not be intimidated by terminology or any time constraints of the professionals. If the meeting can't be finished in the allotted time, it can be continued at a later

date. The importance of this meeting cannot be over-emphasized, so make sure you understand exactly what is happening.

4. Do not sign your agreement with the placement prior to consultation with professionals and your spouse. After the meeting you will be asked to sign several documents. Do not sign anything that says that you approve of the placement at this meeting unless your doctor or other professional is present and agrees with the educational plan. Discuss the placement with your doctor and other professionals, with your spouse, and with your child. Once you have signed this document it becomes much more difficult (but not impossible) to change your child's placement. The only document you should sign is the attendance sheet that indicates your attendance at the meeting. *Read everything before signing.* If you do not understand what you are asked to sign, don't sign it. You can wait, read it carefully at your convenience, discuss it with professionals, and sign it later if you agree with the treatment plan.

What Placements Are Available?

Each school district handles special education services differently. Usually there is a central facility to educate the most severely handicapped children. Other special education programs are usually scattered throughout the school district. Local schools may offer two types of special education placements. In the first type of placement called *mainstreaming with support*, children spend most of their time in a regular classroom and are taken out of the classroom for special instruction such as speech therapy, or educational remediation. The second type of placement is called a *self-contained classroom* situation. In a self-contained classroom, children spend the majority of time in a classroom with only a few students (usually less than 10), all of whom have similar problems. Some children remain in the self-contained classroom for all periods with the exception of lunch and physical education. Other children leave the self-contained classroom at various times to participate in mainstream academic activities or to receive special therapy. In primary schools, the self-contained special education classrooms are usually scattered throughout the various elementary schools in the district. Thus, there might be a second-grade learning disability classroom at one school while the second-grade emotional disability classroom is at another school. Often the professional therapists, such as social workers and speech therapists, visit different schools on different days of the week. A child in a self-contained classroom might have speech therapy on Mondays and Wednesdays, and physical therapy on Tuesdays. Since resources are scarce, it is unlikely that your school district will have full-time specialists for each elementary school in the district.

The educational plan presented to you at the staffing will indicate which placement option (or options) the school district believes is most appropriate for your child. They should offer you the opportunity to observe the particular classroom or teacher being recommended before requiring you to make a decision.

After the staffing, you and your doctor should get together privately to discuss the placement options suggested by the school. If you are satisfied with the placement, you should still meet the teacher and observe the classroom. If, after discussing the placement with your doctor and other professionals, visiting the teachers, and observing the classrooms, you are satisfied with the placement, then it is time to sign the papers agreeing to the placement.

What If You Disagree with the Placement?

Perhaps, after visiting the suggested placement, you do not feel that it is appropriate for your child. Since you have not yet given your consent to the placement you can ask for another meeting to try to convince the school district to offer a different placement. Your course of action at this time will depend on your reasons for disagreeing with the placement. The following sections deal with the most common reasons parents reject a placement.

1. "I don't want my child stigmatized by being in a learning disability classroom." This reason is the most common, and it is the easiest to deal with. Children with special educational needs suffer more emotional harm from being inappropriately in a mainstream classroom than from the "stigma" of being in a self-contained classroom. It is much more important for your child to receive the emotional and academic support of an appropriate placement than to avoid the stigma with the placement. So I do not view this as a valid reason to reject a placement.

2. "I agree with the placement decision but am not pleased about the location of the classroom or the particular teacher." Depending on the size of the school district, there may be a different classroom or teacher available for your child. Most school districts have no trouble agreeing to a request such as this one.

In small districts there may be no alternatives. Rarely, the district may be willing to place your child in another school district or even a private program. In that event, the district must pay for these services, so they are usually reluctant to admit they do not have an appropriate placement available for your child. You may come to an impasse. How to handle an impasse is discussed later in this chapter.

3. "I disagree with the conclusions of the school's evaluation of my child's handicaps." This is an important problem. Perhaps the school has suggested an emotional disability classroom and you believe a learning disability classroom is a better choice or vice versa. If this is the case, you need to discuss the issues with other professionals and your doctor. If these consultants agree with your assessment (namely, that the conclusion of the school is wrong) you can ask for another meeting where you can present evidence (letters from doctors, teachers, and therapists, testimony from professionals, etc.) in an attempt to convince the school of their error. If there is evidence that they have made a misjudgment, most school districts will agree to try the placement you and your doctor suggest. If the school district is not convinced by your argument and refuse to alter their recommendation, you have reached an impasse.

How Do I Proceed If I Reach an Impasse with the School District?

If you and the school district come to an impasse, you have two choices. The first is to enroll your child in a private school. Parents have more control of placement and services in private schools than in public schools. The school may have the necessary ancillary services, such as PT, OT, speech therapy, etc., or you may have to pay private professionals to provide these services at home or at school. Obviously, this is extremely expensive.

If private school is not an alternative, then your next recourse is to request a due process hearing. This is your legal right. Due process hearings are legal proceedings and require lawyers, depositions, etc., and can be extremely costly and time-consuming. Before proceeding to a due process hearing, make sure you can call on professionals to support your position. The opinion of a parent will not be given the same weight as that of a doctor or professional therapist. It is also a good idea to keep in mind that the school district wants the same thing for your child as you do—the best possible placement and the best possible outcome for the child. Again, issues of stigmatization should not be a consideration at this point. You should weigh the alternatives carefully before proceeding. My suggestion is that unless you and your consultants strongly believe that the suggested placement will be detrimental to your child, give the school district's placement a try. Then, after your child has been in the classroom for a few months, if you still feel the placement is inappropriate or inadequate, you can ask for another staffing to reassess the placement. At this point your child's teacher will have new input into how he or she is adapting to the classroom.

Since it can take a handicapped child several months to adapt to a new placement, I suggest waiting at least six months before asking for another staffing.

Try to keep an open mind about your child's placement. Don't sabotage your child's chances by allowing him or her to sense your disapproval of the placement.

What Happens after the Placement?

In the spring, another staffing will be held to discuss the next year's placement and programs for your child. Formal testing is not usually performed annually. I think it is a good idea to repeat educational testing at least every two years. As children grow, new strengths or weaknesses may become evident. As in the original placement staffing, both parents should participate and it is a good idea to have a professional accompany you to the annual staffing, to act as an interpreter and to help you understand the reasons behind the conclusions and placement recommendations.

A final reminder: you and the school districts have the same goals, the best education for your child. On the other hand they have limited financial resources available to them. You, with the help of your doctor and other professionals, must take an active role to assure that the best possible treatment plan has been developed for your child. For example, if your doctor feels your child needs speech therapy and the district has no speech therapist, you may need a due process hearing to force the school district to pay for a private therapist. It is a difficult task, but you have the ultimate responsibility for your child. Do not abrogate this responsibility to the school district.

Try to work *with* the school district, but fight them if you have to in order to get the best possible services for your child.

Caring for handicapped children requires the coordinated efforts of parents and professionals. Parents must take active roles in choosing professionals and making therapeutic decisions. Raising a handicapped child requires a tremendous amount of effort. By using all the resources available, parents can successfully provide the necessary services for their handicapped child and maintain their personal and family life. I hope this book has been a helpful guide in your efforts towards accomplishing this goal.

Listing of National Support Groups and Voluntary Organizations

Abstracted from: *A Guide to National Genetic Voluntary Organizations* (January 1989) and *A Directory of National Organizations Related to Maternal and Child Health* (March 1989), published by the National Center for Education in Maternal and Child Health. Free copies of these publications can be obtained by contacting the NCEMCH at 38th and R Streets, NW, Washington, D.C. 20057, telephone 202-625-8400.

GENERAL GENETICS AND BIRTH DEFECTS

Alliance of Genetic Support
  Groups
38th and R Streets, NW
Washington, DC 20057
(202) 625-7853

March of Dimes Birth Defects
  Foundation
1275 Mamaroneck Ave.
White Plains, NY 10605
(914) 428-7100

National Easter Seal Society
2023 West Ogden Ave.
Chicago, IL 60612
(312) 243-8400

National Foundation for Jewish
Genetic Diseases, Inc.
250 Park Ave.
Suite 1000
New York, NY 10177
(212) 682-5550

National Organization for Rare
Disorders, Inc.
PO Box 8923
New Fairfield, CT 06812
(800) 447-6673
(203) 746-6518

Sibling Information Network
University Affiliated Program
on Developmental Disabilities
University of Connecticut
249 Glenbrook Road
Box U-64
Storrs, CT 06268
(203) 486-3783

The Association for Persons
with Severe Handicaps
7010 Roosevelt Way, NE
Seattle, WA 98115
(206) 523-8446

AUDITORY

Alexander Graham Bell Association for the Deaf (AGBAD)
3417 Volta Place, NW
Washington, DC 20007
(202) 337-5220

American Society for Deaf Children (ASDC)
814 Thayer Ave.
Silver Spring, MD 20910
(301) 585-5400

CHROMOSOMAL

Association for Children with
Down Syndrome, Inc.
(ACDS)
2616 Martin Ave.
Bellmore
Long Island, NY 11710
(516) 221-4700

5p- Society (Cri du Chat or
Cat Cry Syndrome Support
Group)
11609 Oakmont
Overland Park, KS 66210
(913) 469-8900

Fragile X Foundation
PO Box 300233
Denver, CO 80203
(800) 835-2246 ext. 58

Fragile X Support, Inc.
1380 Huntington Drive
Mundelein, IL 60060
(312) 680-3317

National Association for Down
Syndrome (NADS)
PO Box 4542
Oakbrook, IL 60521
(312) 325-9112

National Down Syndrome Congress (NDSC) (Resources and Support Group)
1800 Dempster St.
Park Ridge, IL 60068-1146
(312) 823-7550
(800) 232-NDSC (Outside Illinois)

National Down Syndrome Society (NDSS)
141 Fifth Avenue
Suite 75
New York, NY 10010
(212) 460-9330
(800) 221-4602

Prader-Willi Syndrome Association (PWSA)
6490 Excelsior Blvd.
E-102
St. Louis Park, MN
(612) 926-1947

Support Group for Monosomy 9P
43304 Kipton Nickel Plate Road
La Grange, OH 44050
(216) 775-4255

Support Organization for Trisomy 18, 13 and Other Related Disorders
(S.O.F.T. 18/13)
5030 Cole
Pocatello, ID 83202
(208) 237-8782

CONNECTIVE TISSUE

National Marfan Foundation (NMF)
382 Main St.
Port Washington, NY 11050
(516) 838-8712

DEVELOPMENTAL DISABILITIES

Association for Children and Adults with Learning Disabilities, Inc. (ACLD)
4156 Library Road
Pittsburgh, PA 15234
(412) 341-1515

Association for Retarded Citizens of the United States (ARC)
2501 Avenue J
Arlington, TX 76006
(817) 640-0204

Autism Society of America (ASA)
1234 Massachusetts Ave., NW
Suite 1017
Washington, DC 20005-4599
(202) 783-0215

Lawrence-Moon-Biedl Syn-
  drome (LMBS) Support Network (Bardet-Biedl)
122 Rolling Road
Lexington Park, MD 20653
(301)863-5658

Orton Dyslexia Society (ODS)
724 York Road
Baltimore, MD 21204
(301) 296-0232

Progeria International Registry
New York State Institute for
  Basic Research
Department of Human Genetics
1050 Forest Hill Road
Staten Island, NY 10314
(718) 494-5230

Rubenstein-Taybi Syndrome
  (RTS) Parent Group
414 East Kansas
Smith Center, KS 66967
(913) 282-6237

Share and Care (Support
  Group for families of children with Cockayne
Syndrome)
1294 "S" St.
North Valley Stream, NY 11580
(516) 825-2284

United Cerebral Palsy Associa-
  tions, Inc. (UCPA) / UCP
  Research and
Educational Foundation
66 East 34th St.
New York, NY 10016
(212) 481-6300
(800) USA-1UCP

MENTAL HEALTH

Depression and Related Affective Disorders, Inc. (DRADA)
John Hopkins Hospital
Meyer 4-181
601 North Wolfe St.
Baltimore, MD 21205
(301) 955-3246

METABOLIC

American Porphyria Foundation
PO Box 11163
Montgomery, AL 36111
(205) 265-2200

Association for Glycogen Storage Disease
Box 896
Durant, IA 52747
(319) 785-6038

Association of Neuro-Metabolic
  Disorders
5223 Brookfield Lane
Sylvania, OH 43560
(419) 885-1497

Dysautonomia Foundation, Inc.
370 Lexington Ave.
New York, NY 10017
(212) 889-5222

Foundation for the Study of
  Wilson's Disease, Inc.
5447 Palisade Ave.
Bronx, NY 10471
(212) 430-2091

Lowe's Syndrome Association,
Inc.
222 Lincoln St.
West Lafayette, ID 47906
(317) 743-3634

Maple Syrup Urine Disease
(MSUD) Family Support
Group
R.R. #2
Box 24-A
Flemingsburg, KY 41041
(606) 849-4679

ML (Mucolipidosis) IV Foundation
6 Concord Drive
Monsey, NY 10952
(919) 425-0639

National Gaucher Foundation,
Inc. (NGF)
1424 "K" St., NW
Fourth Floor
Washington, DC 20005
(202) 393-2777

National Mucopolysaccharidoses
(MPS) Society, Inc.
17 Kraemer St.
Hicksville, NY 11801
(516) 931-6338

National Tay-Sachs and Allied
Diseases Association, Inc.
(NTSAD)
385 Elliot St.
Newton, MA 02164
(617) 964-5508

Organic Acidemia Association,
Inc.
1532 South 87 St.
Kansas City, KS 66111
(913) 422-7080

United Leukodystrophy Foundation, Inc. (ULF)
2304 Highland Drive
Sycamore, IL 60178
(815) 895-3211

Williams Syndrome Association
(WSA)
PO Box 178373
San Diego, CA 2117-0910
(713) 376-7072

Wilson's Disease Association
PO Box 75324
Washington, DC 20013
(703) 636-3003,3014

Zain Hansen M.P.S.
(Mucopolysaccaridosis) Foundation
PO Box 4768
1200 Fernwood Drive
Arcata, CA 95521
(707) 822-5421

NEUROLOGIC

Alzheimer's Disease and Related Disorders Association,
Inc. (ADRDA)
70 East Lake St.
Chicago, IL 60601
(312) 853-3060
(800) 631-0379

Batten's Disease Support and
  Research Association
6707 197th St. East
Spanaway, WA 98387
(206) 847-2926

Epilepsy Foundation of America
  (EFA)
4351 Garden City Drive
Landover, MD 20785
(301) 459-3700

Friedreich's Ataxia Group in
  America (FAGA)
PO Box 1116
Oakland, CA 94611
(415) 655-0833

Hereditary Disease Foundation
  (biomedical research on
  Huntington's disease and
  other neurological illnesses)
606 Wilshire Blvd.
Suite 504
Santa Monica, CA 90401-9990
(213) 458-4183

Huntington's Disease Society of
  America, Inc. (HDSA)
140 West 22nd St.
New York, NY 10011-2420
(212) 242-1968

International Joseph Diseases
  Foundation, Inc. (LJDF)
PO Box 2550
Livermore, CA 94550

International Rett Syndrome Association, Inc. (IRSA)
8511 Rose Mare Drive
Fort Washington, MD 20744
(301) 248-7031

National Hydrocephalus Founda-
  tion (NHF)
Route 1
River Road
Box 210 A
Joliet, IL 60436
(815) 467-6548

National Neurofibromatosis
  Foundation, Inc.
141 Fifth Ave.
Suite 7-S
New York, NY 10010
(212) 460-8980
(800) 323-7983

National Tuberous Sclerosis Association, Inc. (NTSA)
4351 Garden City Drive
Suite 660
Landover, MD 20785
(301) 459-9888
(800) CAL-NTSA

Spina Bifida Association of
  America (SBAA)
1700 Rockville Pike
Suite 540
Rockville, MD 20852
(301) 770-7222
(800) 621-3141

Sturge-Weber Foundation
  (Sturge-Weber Syndrome)
PO Box 460931
Aurora, CO 80015
(303) 693-2986

Tourette Syndrome Association, Inc. (TSA)
42-40 Bell Blvd.
Bayside, NY 11361
(718) 224-2999

Tuberous Sclerosis Association of America (TSSA)
PO Box 1305
Middleboro, MA 02370
(617) 947-8893

NEUROMUSCULAR

Amyotrophic Lateral Sclerosis Association, Inc. (ALSA)
(Lou Gehrig's disease)
15300 Ventura Boulevard
Suite 315
Sherman Oaks, California 91403
(818) 990-2151

AVENUES - National Support Group for Arthrogryposis Multiplex Congenita
PO Box 5192
Sonora, CA 95370
(209) 928-3689

CMT (Charcot-Marie-Tooth) International, Inc. (peroneal muscular atrophy and hereditary motor and sensory neuropathy)
34 Bayview Drive
St. Catharines
Ontario L2N 4Y6
Canada
(416) 937-3851

Dystonia Medical Research Foundation (DMRF)
8383 Wilshire Blvd.
Suite 800
Beverly Hills, CA 90210
(213) 852-1630

Families of S.M.A. (Spinal Muscular Atrophy)
PO Box 1465
Highland Park, IL 60035
(312) 432-5551

Muscular Dystrophy Association (MDA)
810 Seventh Ave.
New York, NY 10019
(212) 586-0808

Myasthenia Gravis Foundation, Inc. (MGF)
7-11 South Broadway
Suite 304
White Plains, NY 10601
(914) 328-1717

Myoclonus Families United
1564 East 34th St.
Brooklyn, NY 11234
(718) 252-2133

National Ataxia Foundation
600 Twelve Oaks Center
15500 Wayzata Blvd.
Wayzata, MN 55391
(612) 473-7666

National Multiple Sclerosis Society
205 East 42nd St.
New York, NY 10017
(212) 986-3240

SKIN

Xeroderma Pigmentosum Registry
UMDNJ
New Jersy Medical School Department of Pathology
Room C-520
Medical Science Building
100 Bergen St.
Newark, NJ 07103
(201) 456-6255

VISUAL

American Foundation for the
  Blind, Inc. (AFB)
15 West 16th St.
New York, NY 10011
(212) 620-2000

Blind Children's Fund
230 Central St.
Auburndale, MA 02166-2399
(617) 332-4014

National Association for Parents
  of the Visually Impaired, Inc.
(NAPVI)
PO Box 180806
Austin, TX 78718
(512) 323-5710

National Association for Visually Handicapped
22 West 21st St.
Sixth Floor
New York, NY 10010
(212) 889-3141

Retinitis Pigmentosum Foundation Fighting Blindness
National Headquarters
1401 Mount Royale Ave., 4th floor
Baltimore, MD, 21217
Toll free: 800-638-2300
In Baltimore: 301-225-9400

Smith-Lemli-Opitz Syndrome
5 Hampton Court
Newark, DE 19703
(302) 834-4157

Parents of Galactosemic Children, Inc.
One Ash Court
New City, NY 10956
(914) 638-3650

Children's Brain Diseases Foundation
350 Parnassus Ave.
Suite 900
San Francisco, CA 94117
(415) 566-5402

Federation for Children with
  Special Needs
312 Stuart St.
Second floor
Boston, MA 02116
(617) 482-2915

National Parent CHAIN (Coalition for Handicapped Americans Information Network)
90 East Wilson Bridge Road
Suite 297
Worthington, OH 43085
(614) 431-1911

REHABILITATION

American Occupational Therapy
  Association, Inc. (AOTA)
1383 Piccard Drive
Suite 301
Rockville, MD 20850
(301) 948-9626

American Physical Therapy Association (APTA)
111 North Fairfax St.
Alexandria, VA 22314
(703) 684-2782

Council of State Administrators
  of Vocational Rehabilitation
PO Box 3776
Washington, DC 20007
(202) 638-4634

National Easter Seal Society
2023 West Ogden Ave.
Chicago, IL 60612
(312) 243-8400

National Rehabilitation Association
633 South Washington St.
Alexandria, VA 22313
(703) 836-0850

National Rehabilitation Information Center (NRIC)
8455 Colesville Road
Suite 935
Silver Spring, MD 20910-3319
(301) 588-9284

SPECIAL EDUCATION

American Council on Rural Spe-
  cial Education (ACRES)
Miller Hall 359
Western Washington University
Bellingham, WA 98225
(206) 676-3576

Council for Exceptional Children (CEC)
1920 Association Drive
Reston, VA 22091
(703) 620-3660

National Association of State
  Directors of Special Education (NASDSE)
2021 "K" St., NW
Suite 315
Washington, DC 20006
(202) 296-1800

National Information Center
  for Children and Youth with
  Handicaps (NICHCY)
PO Box 1492
Washington, DC 20013
(703) 893-6061

Glossary

ADD: Attention deficit disorder.

ADD-H: Attention deficit disorder with hyperactivity.

Age equivalent: The age at which a given test score would be in the 50th percentile.

Allele: One of the two genes present in each individual for autosomal traits.

Anticonvulsant: A medicine used to prevent epileptic seizures.

Apgar test: A test that assesses the condition of a newborn infant. A score of 10 is the best score, a score of 0 is the worst score.

Asphyxia: Any process depriving oxygen to the brain.

Attention deficit disorder (ADD): An individual who has difficulty concentrating on tasks.

Attention deficit disorder with hyperactivity (ADD-H): An individual with ADD in addition to problems with excessive movements (hyperactivity).

Amniocentesis: A technique for prenatal diagnosis performed in the fourth month of pregnancy.

Autism: Severe disability involving relating to others and speech.

Autosome: Any of the 22 pairs of chromosomes that are not sex chromosomes.

Autosomal dominant genetic disease: a disease caused by the presence of a single abnormal gene.

Autosomal recessive genetic disease: A disease caused by the presence of 2 abnormal genes.

Bases: The four chemical building blocks that make up DNA.

Brain stem: The area of the brain controlling unconscious actions.

Brazelton examination: a special physical examination of infants that assesses cortical brain function.

Chorionic villus sampling: A technique for prenatal diagnosis performed in the second–third month of pregnancy.

Chromosomal disease: Disease due to abnormal amounts or structure of chromosomes.

Chromosomes: Structures visible under a microscope that contain all the genes of an individual.

Codon: A sequence of three base pairs forming a genetic word. A single codon can code for "start," "stop" or one of the 20 amino acids used in making protein.

Decreased muscle tone: See hypotonia.

Deletion: Abnormal chromosome structure in which material from one of the chromosomes has been lost.

DNA: Deoxyribonucleic acid. The chemical substance that genes and chromosomes are made of.

Developmental milestones: Skills obtained by children during infancy, toddlerhood, and childhood, i.e., walking, talking, stacking blocks.

Developmental testing: Tests administered to infants to assess their achievement of developmental milestones.

Dyslexia: Brain dysfunction resulting in partial-to-complete impairment in the ability to read.

Dysmorphic: The presence of a peculiar structure or appearance in an individual.

Dysmorphology: The study of children with birth defects.

Educational testing: A battery of tests designed to assess function with respect to learning and acquiring cognitive skills.

Educational therapy: A discipline specializing in optimizing learning for children with mental retardation and learning disabilities.

Emotional disability (ED): An individual whose primary problem is felt to involve social and psychological dysfunction.

Five minute Apgar score: The results of an Apgar test performed at 5 minutes of age.

Fragile X syndrome: X-linked genetic disease causing mental retardation and autistic-like symptoms.

Gene: A piece of DNA containing the information for a particular trait.

Genetic: Involving the hereditary elements (genes and chromosomes).

Genetic code: The genetic "dictionary" specifying the meaning of each codon.

Genetic counseling: The process of determining if an individual or couple is at risk for having a child with a genetic disease or multiple malformation syndrome.

Genetic disease: Disease whose primary causation is due to the genetic makeup of the individual.

Geneticist: Physician specializing in the diagnosis and treatment of genetic diseases and multiple malformation syndromes.

Grade equivalent: The grade at which a given score would be in the 50th percentile.

Hemizygous: Describes the status of a man for any X-linked gene.

Heterozygous: The state in which both genes for a given trait are different.

Homozygous: The state in which both genes for a particular trait are identical.

Hypertonia: The presence of increased muscle tone. The muscles are rigid and spastic.

Hypotonia: The presence of decreased muscle tone. The muscles seem weak and flaccid.

IEP: See Individual Educational Plan.

Inborn error of metabolism: Inherited metabolic disease.

Increased muscle tone: See hypertonia.

Individual Educational Plan (IEP): A school district plan for the education, placement, and therapies for a handicapped child.

Inherited metabolic disease: One of several genetic diseases resulting from an inability to carry out one or more of the chemical reactions in the body.

Inversion: An abnormality of chromosome structure in which a piece of the chromosome breaks off, flips around, and reattaches in the wrong orientation.

IQ: Intelligence quotient. A standardized measurement of intellectual functioning.

Karyotype: Analysis of an individual's chromosomal content.

LD: See Learning disability.

Learning disability (LD): An individual with a normal IQ who is unable to function well in a mainstream classroom and whose educational testing reveals specific areas of deficit.

Lysosomes: The cellular elements responsible for the breakdown of cellular debris.

Lysosomal storage disease: An inherited metabolic disease involving dysfunctional lysosomes.

Mean: Average.

Median: The number at which there is an equal number above and an equal number below.

Metabolic disease: Inherited metabolic disease.

Mosaic: An individual containing more than one genetic type of cell.

Multiple malformation syndrome: A combination of birth defects which occur together. These can be genetic or nongenetic in etiology.

Neurologist: A physician specializing in the diagnosis and treatment of diseases affecting the brain, nerves, and muscles.

Occupational therapy: A discipline which specializes in helping individuals adapt to their handicap for optimum functioning.

One minute Apgar score: The results of an Apgar test at one minute of age.

Organic acidemias: A family of inherited metabolic diseases caused by inability to properly digest protein.

Pediatric neurologist: A neurologist specialized in the care of children with disorders affecting the brain, nerves, and muscles.

Percentile: A test score that indicates how many individuals scored above and how many individuals scored below a given child's score. (The 50th percentile equals the median.)

Perinatal: Pertaining to events surrounding labor and delivery and the immediate newborn period.

Perinatal asphyxia: Deprivation of oxygen to a baby's brain during labor, delivery, and/or the immediate newborn period.

Physical therapy: A discipline which specializes in training and rehabilitation of physical handicaps and injuries.

Psychological testing: A battery of tests designed to assess psychological, psychiatric, social, and/or educational functioning.

Psychology: A broad discipline which encompasses psychotherapy, developmental specialties, and special training to administer psychological and/or educational testing.

Raw test score: A test score which has not been standardized.

Respite care: A service provided for parents of handicapped children where a child lives for several days to a few weeks in a facility staffed by trained professionals.

Sex chromosomes: The one pair of chromosomes (2) involved in sex determination (X chromosome and the Y chromosome).

Seizure disorder: Epilepsy.

Spastic: Muscles that are stiff and difficult to move.

Sex-linked genetic disease: See X-linked genetic disease.

Staffing: A meeting in a school or other facility where teachers, aides, social workers, psychologists, and therapists discuss the progress and plan for a child.

Standardized test score: A test result reported in terms of how an individual compares to a population group.

Teratogen: An agent which is capable of causing birth defects.

Teratology: The study of teratogens.

X-linked genetic disease: A disease caused by a defective gene on the X chromosome.

Bibliography

Books: General Genetics

Strom, CM. *Have a Healthy Baby*, Prentice-Hall, Englewood Cliffs, 1988.

This book is for the lay public and contains chapters on genetics and birth defects.

Thompson, JS, Thompson, MW. *Genetics in Medicine*, 4th ed., W.B. Saunders, Philadelphia, 1986.

A good basic human genetics text suitable for individuals with a college biology background.

McKusick, VA. *Mendelian Inheritance in Man*, 7th ed., Johns Hopkins University Press, Baltimore, 1986.

This book is the encyclopedic compendium of all genetic disorders. You will need a medical dictionary to use this book, and probably help from a physician.

Emery, AE, Rimoin, DL. *Principles and Practice of Medical Genetics*, Churchill Livingstone, New York, 1983.

This book is the definitive genetics textbook for physicians.

Jones, KL. *Smith's Recognizable Patterns of Human Malformation*, 4th ed., W.B. Saunders, Philadelphia, 1988.

This is the definitive compendium of multiple malformation syndromes. Contains pictures and descriptions of each syndrome and is indexed by abnormality. You will need a medical dictionary to use this book.

Scriver, CR, Beaudet, AL, Sly, WS, Valle, D. *The Metabolic Basis of Inherited Disease*, 6th ed., McGraw-Hill, New York, 1989.

The definitive text (in 2 volumes) describing in detail all inborn errors of metabolism (metabolic diseases).

Articles

Incidence of Genetic Diseases

Baird, PA, Anderson, TW, Newcombe, HB *et al.* Genetic disorders in children and young adults: A population study, *Am. J. Hum. Genet.*, 42:677–693, 1988.

Laws to Provide Services to Handicapped Children

Wright, GF. The pediatrician's role in Public Law 94-142, *Pediatrics in Rev.*, 4:191–197, 1982.

Meyen, EL, Public Law 94-142: Comments on the pediatricians contribution from an educator, *Pediatrics*, 491–494, 1982.

Wilson's Disease

Cartwright, GE, Diagnosis of treatable Wilson's disease, *New Engl. J. of Med.*, 298:1347–1350, 1978.

Autism and Rett's Syndrome

Matsuishi, T, Shiotsuki, Y, Niikawa, N, Katafuchi, Y et al. Fragile X syndrome in Japanese patients with infantile autism, *Pediatr. Neurol.* 3(5):284–7, 1987.

Sanua, VD. Studies in infantile autism. *Child Psychiatry Hum. Dev.* 19(3):207–27, 1989.

Howlin, P. Living with impairment: The effects on children of having an autistic sibling, *Child Care Health Dev.* 14(6):395–408, 1988.

Minshew, NJ, Payton, JB. New perspectives in autism, Part I: The clinical spectrum of autism, *Curr. Probl. Pediatr.* 18(10):561–610, 1988.

Leboyer, M, Osherson, DN, Nosten, M, Roubertoux, P. Is autism associated with anomalous dominance? *J. Autism Dev. Disord.* 18(4):539–51, 1988.

Minshew, NJ, Payton, JB. New perspectives in autism, Part II: The differential diagnosis and neurobiology of autism, *Curr. Probl. Pediatr.* 18(11):613–94, 1988.

Naidu, S, Kitt, CA, Wong, DF, Price, DL, et al. Research on Rett syndrome: Strategy and preliminary results, *J. Child Neurol.* 3 Suppl:S78–86, 1988.

Zoghbi, H. Genetic aspects of Rett syndrome, *J. Child Neurol.* 3 Suppl:S76–8, 1988.

Percy AK. Research in Rett syndrome: Past, present, and future, *J. Child Neurol.* 3 Suppl:S72–5, 1988.

Rimland B. Controversies in the treatment of autistic children: Vitamin and drug therapy, *J. Child Neurol.* 3 Suppl:S68–72, 1988.

Trevathan E; Naidu S. The clinical recognition and differential diagnosis of Rett syndrome, *J. Child Neurol.* 3 Suppl:S6–16, 1988.

Schreibman L. Diagnostic features of autism, *J. Child Neurol.* 3 Suppl:S57–64, 1988.

Lieb-Lundell, C. The therapist's role in the management of girls with Rett syndrome, *J. Child Neurol.* 3 Suppl:S31–4, 1988.

Trevathan, E, Adams, MJ. The epidemiology and public health significance of Rett syndrome, *J. Child Neurol.* 3 Suppl:S17–20, 1988.

Burd, L, Gascon, GG. Rett syndrome: Review and discussion of current diagnostic criteria, *J. Child Neurol.* 3(4):263–8, 1988.

Rapin, I. Disorders of higher cerebral function in preschool children, Second of two parts, *Am. J. Dis. Child* 142(11):1178–82, 1988.

Baron-Cohen, S. Social and pragmatic deficits in autism: Cognitive or affective? *J. Autism Dev. Disord.* 18(3):379–402, 1988.

Smalley, SL, Asarnow, RF, Spence, MA. Autism and genetics. A decade of research, *Arch. Gen. Psychiatry* 45(10):953–61, 1988.

Gillberg, C. The neurobiology of infantile autism, *J. Child Psychol. Psychiatry* 29(3):257–66, 1988.

du Verglas, G, Banks, SR, Guyer, KE. Clinical effects of fenfluramine on children with autism: A review of the research, *J. Autism Dev. Disord.* 18(2):297–308, 1988.

Morgan, SB. The autistic child and family functioning: A developmental-family systems perspective, *J. Autism Dev. Disord.* 18(2):263–80, 1988.

Feinstein, C, Kaminer, Y, Barrett, RP, Tylenda, B. The assessment of mood and affect in developmentally disabled children and adolescents: The Emotional Disorders Rating Scale, *Res. Dev. Disabil.* 9(2):109–21, 1988.

Allen, DA, Rapin, I, Wiznitzer, M. Communication disorders of preschool children: The physician's responsibility, *J. Dev. Behav. Pediatr.* 9(3):164–70, 1988.

Moeschler, JB, Charman, CE, Berg, SZ, Graham, JM Jr. Rett syndrome: Natural history and management, *Pediatrics* 82(1):1–10, 1988.

Campbell, M, Spencer, EK. Psychopharmacology in child and adolescent psychiatry: A review of the past five years, *J. Am. Acad. Child Adolesc. Psychiatry* 27(3):269–79, 1988.

Folstein, SE, Rutter, ML. Autism: Familial aggregation and genetic implications, *J. Autism Dev. Disord.* 18(1):3–30, 1988.

Campbell, M. Fenfluramine treatment of autism, *J. Child Psychol. Psychiatry* 29(1):1–10, 1988.

Learning Disabilities

Chalfant, JC. Learning disabilities. Policy issues and promising approaches, *Am. Psychol.* 44(2):392–8, 1989.

Shaywitz, SE, Shaywitz, BA. Attention deficit disorder: Current perspectives, *Pediatr. Neurol.* 3(3):129–35, 1987.

Schunk, DH. Self-efficacy and cognitive achievement: implications for students with learning problems, *J. Learn. Disabil.* 22(1):14–22, 1989.

Grande, G. *Educational Therapy for the Failing and Frustrated Student Offender.*

Coplin, JW, Morgan, SB. Learning disabilities: A multidimensional perspective, *J. Learn. Disabil.* 21(10):614–22, 1988.

Stanovich, KE. Explaining the differences between the dyslexic and the garden-variety poor reader: The phonological-core variable-difference model. *J. Learn. Disabil.* 21(10):590–604, 1988.

Gordon, BN, Jens, KG. A conceptual model for tracking high-risk infants and making early service decisions, *J. Dev. Behav. Pediatr.* 9(5):279–86, 1988.

Ceci, SJ, Baker, JG. On learning ... more or less: A knowledge x process x context view of learning disabilities, *J. Learn. Disabil.* 22(2):90–9, 1989.

Ault, MJ, Wolery, M, Doyle, PM, Gast, DL. Review of comparative studies in the instruction of students with moderate and severe handicaps, *Except. Child* 55(4):346–56, 1989.

Spreen, O. Prognosis of learning disability, *J. Consult. Clin. Psychol.* 56(6):836–42, 1988.

Lyon, GR, Moats, LC. Critical issues in the instruction of the learning disabled. *J. Consult. Clin. Psychol.* 56(6):830–5, 1988.

Satz P, Fletcher, JM. Early identification of learning disabled children: An old problem revisited, *J. Consult. Clin. Psychol.* 56(6):824–9, 1988.

Pennington, BF, Smith, SD. Genetic influences on learning disabilities: An update, *J. Consult. Clin. Psychol.* 56(6):817–23, 1988.

Rourke, BP. Socioemotional disturbances of learning-disabled children, *J. Consult. Clin. Psychol.* 56(6):801–10, 1988.

Taylor, HG. Neuropsychological testing: Relevance for assessing children's learning disabilities, *J. Consult. Clin. Psychol.* 56(6):795–800, 1988.

Morris, RD. Classification of learning disabilities: old problems and new approaches. *J. Consult. Clin. Psychol.* 56(6):789–94, 1988.

Klerman, LV. School absence—A health perspective, *Pediatr. Clin. North Am.* 35(6):1253–69, 1988.

Palfrey, JS, Rappaport, LA. School placement, *Pediatr. Rev.* 8(9):261–71, 1987.

Larson, KA. A research review and alternative hypothesis explaining the link between learning disability and delinquency, *J. Learn. Disabil.* 21(6):357–63, 369, 1988.

Grande, CG. Delinquency: The learning disabled student's reaction to academic school failure? *Adolescence* 23(89):209–19, 1988.

McGee, R, Share, DL. Attention deficit disorder-hyperactivity and academic failure: Which comes first and what should be treated? *J. Am. Acad. Child Adolesc. Psychiatry* (3):318–25, 1988.

Werry, JS. Drugs, learning and cognitive function in children—an update, *J. Child Psychol. Psychiatry* 29(2):129–41, 1988.

Forness, SR, Kavale, KA. Psychopharmacologic treatment: A note on classroom effects, *J. Learn. Disabil.* 21(3):144–7, 1988.

Woodward, JP, Carnine, DW. Antecedent knowledge and intelligent computer assisted instruction, *J. Learn. Disabil.* 21(3):131–9, 1988.

Loehlin, JC, Willerman, L. Horn JM. Human behavior genetics, *Annu. Rev. Psychol.* 39:101–33, 1988.

Bryan, T, Bay, M, Donahue M. Implications of the learning disabilities definition for the regular education initiative, *J. Learn. Disabil.* 21(1):23–8, 1988.

Decker, SN, Bender, BG. Converging evidence for multiple genetic forms of reading disability, *Brain Lang.* 33(2):197–215, 1988.

Tourette Syndrome

Adkins, AS. Helping your patient cope with Tourette syndrome. *Pediatr. Nurs.* 15(2):135–7, 1989.

Messiha, FS. Biochemical pharmacology of Gilles de la Tourette's syndrome, *Neurosci. Biobehav. Rev.* 12(3–4):295–305, 1988.

Kerbeshian, J, Burd, L. A clinical pharmacological approach to treating Tourette syndrome in children and adolescents, *Neurosci. Biobehav. Rev.* 12(3–4):241-5, 1988.

Tardo, C. Tics and Tourette syndrome, *Semin. Neurol.* 8(1):78–82. 1988.

Pennington, BF, Smith, SD. Genetic influences on learning disabilities: an update, *J. Consult. Clin. Psychol.* 56(6):817–23, 1988.

Golden, GS. Tic disorders in childhood, *Pediatr. Rev.* 8(8):229–34, 1987.

Clementz, GL, Lee, RH, Barclay, AM. Tic disorders of childhood, *Am. Fam. Physician* (2):163–70, 1988.

Barabas, G. Tourette's syndrome: An overview, *Pediatr. Ann.* 17(6):391–3, 1988.

Comings, DE. A controlled study of Tourette syndrome, VII, Summary: A common genetic disorder causing disinhibition of the limbic system, *Am. J. Hum. Genet.* 41(5):839–66, 1987.

Comings, DE, Comings, BG. A controlled study of Tourette syndrome, VI, Early development, sleep problems, allergies, and handedness, *Am. J. Hum. Genet.* 41(5):822–38, 1987.

Comings, BG, Comings, DE. A controlled study of Tourette syndrome, V, Depression and mania, *Am. J. Hum. Genet.* 41(5):804–21, 1987.

Comings, DE, Comings, BG. A controlled study of Tourette syndrome, IV, Obsessions, compulsions, and schizoid behaviors, *Am. J. Hum. Genet.* 41(5):782–803, 1987.

Comings, DE, Comings, BG. A controlled study of Tourette syndrome, III, Phobias and panic attacks, *Am. J. Hum. Genet.* 41(5):761–81, 1987.

Comings, DE, Comings, BG. A controlled study of Tourette syndrome, II, Conduct, *Am. J. Hum. Genet.* (5):742–60, 1987.

Comings, DE, Comings, BG. A controlled study of Tourette syndrome, I, Attention-deficit disorder, learning disorders, and school problems, *Am. J. Hum. Genet.* 41(5):701–41, 1987.

Comings, DE, Comings, BG. Evidence for an X-linked modifier gene affecting the expression of Tourette syndrome and its relevance to the increased frequency of speech, cognitive, and behavioral disorders in males, *Proc. Natl. Acad. Sci. USA* 83(8):2551–5, 1986.

Kerbeshian, J, Burd, L. A clinical pharmacological approach to treating Tourette syndrome in children and adolescents, *Neurosci. Biobehav. Rev.* 12(3–4):241–5, 1988.

Attention Deficit Disorder

Henker, B, Whalen, CK. Hyperactivity and attention deficits, *Am. Psychol.* 44(2):216–23, 1989.

Myers, DA, Claman, L, Oldham DG, Waller DA, et al. The hyperactive child: an update. *Tex. Med.* 85(3):25–31, 1989.

Shaywitz, SE, Shaywitz, BA. Attention deficit disorder: Current perspectives, *Pediatr. Neurol.* 3(3):129–35, 1987.

Coleman, WL, Levine, MD. Attention deficits in adolescence: Description, evaluation, and management, *Pediatr. Rev.* 9(9):287–98, 1988.

Orsulak, PJ, Waller, D. Antidepressant drugs: Additional clinical uses. *J. Fam. Pract.* 28(2):209–16, 1989.

Buttross, S. Disorders of attention and vigilance, *Semin. Neurol.* 8(1):97–107, 1988.

Thorley, G. Adolescent outcome for hyperactive children, *Arch. Dis. Child* 63(10):1181–3, 1988.

Rapin, I. Disorders of higher cerebral function in preschool children, 1, *Am. J. Dis. Child* 142(10):1119–24, 1988.

Morgan, AM. Use of stimulant medications in children, *Am. Fam. Physician* 38(4):197–202, 1988.

Klein, RG. Prognosis of attention deficit disorder and its management of adolescence, *Pediatr. Rev.* 8(7):216–22, 1987.

Shaywitz, SE, Shaywitz, BA. Increased medication use in attention-deficit hyperactivity disorder: Regressive or appropriate? *JAMA* 21;260(15):2270–2, 1988.

Kimball, JG. Hypothesis for prediction of stimulant drug effectiveness utilizing sensory integrative diagnostic methods, *J. Am. Osteopath. Assoc.* 88(6):757–62, 1988.

Biederman, J. Pharmacological treatment of adolescents with affective disorders and attention deficit disorder, *Psychopharmacol. Bull.* 24(1):81–7, 1988.

McGee, R, Share, DL. Attention deficit disorder-hyperactivity and academic failure: Which comes first and what should be treated? *J. Am. Acad. Child Adolesc. Psychiatry* 27(3):318–5, 1988.

Jensen, JB, Garfinkel, BD. Neuroendocrine aspects of attention deficit hyperactivity disorder, *Endocrinol. Metab. Clin. North. Am.* 17(1):111–29, 1988.

Porter, LS. The what, why and how of hyperkinesis: Implications for nursing, *J. Adv. Nurs.* 13(2):229–36, 1988.

Bryan, T, Bay, M, Donahue M. Implications of the learning disabilities

definition for the regular education initiative, *J. Learn. Disabil.*
21(1):23–8, 1988.

Fragile X Syndrome

Matsuishi, T, Shiotsuki, Y, Niikawa, N, Katafuchi, Y, et al. Fragile X
syndrome in Japanese patients with infantile autism, *Pediatr. Neurol.*
3(5):284–7, 1987.

Hagerman, RJ, Sobesky, WE. Psychopathology in fragile X syndrome,
Am. J. Orthopsychiatry 59(1):142–52, 1989.

Brown, WT. The fragile X syndrome, *Neurol. Clin.* 7(1):107–21, 1989.

Cronister, AE, Hagerman, RJ. Fragile X syndrome, *J. Pediatr. Health
Care* 3(1):9–19, 1989.

Butler, MG. Fragile X syndrome: A major cause of X-linked mental
retardation, *Compr. Ther.* 14(7):3–7, 1988.

Fisch, GS, Cohen, IL, Jenkins, EC, Brown, WT. Screening developmentally disabled male populations for fragile X: The effect of sample
size, *Am. J. Med. Genet.* 30(1-2):655–63, 1988.

Connor, JM, Ferguson-Smith, MA. Genetic causes of mental handicap
and opportunities for prevention, *Baillieres Clin. Obstet. Gynaecol.*
2(1):37–54, 1988.

Ho, HZ, Glahn, TJ, Ho, JC. The fragile-X syndrome, *Dev. Med. Child
Neurol.* 30(2):257–61, 1988.

Lachiewicz, A, Harrison, C, Spiridigliozzi, GA, Callanan, NP,
Livermore, J. What is the fragile X syndrome? *N. C. Med. J.*
49(4):203–8, 1988.

Klinefelter's Syndrome

Miller, ME, Sulkes, S. Fire-setting behavior in individuals with Klinefelter syndrome, *Pediatrics* 82(1):115–7, 1988.

Klinefelter's syndrome, *Lancet* 11;1(8598):1316–7, 1988.

Eberle, AJ. Klinefelter syndrome and fire-setting behavior [letter], *Pediatrics* 83(4 Pt 2):649–50, 1989.

Sourial, N, Fenton, F. Testosterone treatment of an XXYY male presenting with aggression: A case report, *Can. J. Psychiatry* 33(9):846–50, 1988.

Filippi, G, Pecile, V, Rinaldi, A, Siniscalco, M. Fragile-X mutation and Klinefelter syndrome: A reappraisal, *Am. J. Med. Genet.* 30(1-2):99–107, 1988.

Fryns, JP, Van den Berghe, H. The concurrence of Klinefelter syndrome and fragile X syndrome, *Am. J. Med. Genet.* 30(1-2):109–13, 1988.

Sheridan, MK, Radlinski, S. Brief report: A case study of an adolescent male with XXXXY Klinefelter's syndrome, *J. Autism Dev. Disord.* 18(3):449–56, 1988.

Miller, ME, Sulkes, S. Fire-setting behavior in individuals with Klinefelter syndrome, *Pediatrics* 82(1):115–7, 1988.

Graham, JM Jr, Bashir, AS, Stark, RE, Silbert, A, Walzer, S. Oral and written language abilities of XXY boys: Implications for anticipatory guidance, *Pediatrics* 81(6):795–806, 1988.

Porter, ME, Gardner, HA, DeFeudis, P, Endler, NS. Verbal deficits in Klinefelter (XXY) adults living in the community, *Clin. Genet.* 33(4):246–53, 1988.

Nielsen, J, Pelsen, B. Follow-up 20 years later of 34 Klinefelter males with karyotype 47,XXY and 16 hypogonadal males with karyotype 46,XY, *Hum. Genet.* 77(2):188–92, 1987.

Muller, N, Endres, M. An XX male with schizophrenia: A case of personality development and illness similar to that in XXY males, *J. Clin. Psychiatry* 48(9):379–80, 1987.

Netley, C. Predicting intellectual functioning in 47,XXY boys from characteristics of sibs, *Clin. Genet.* 32(1):24–7, 1987.

Zastowny, TR, Lehman, AF, Dickerson, F. Klinefelter's syndrome and psychopathology: A case study of the combined effects of nature and nurture. *Int. J. Psychiatry Med.* 17(2):155–62, 1987.

Pueschel, SM, O'Brien, MM, Padre-Mendoza, T. Klinefelter syndrome and associated fragile-X syndrome, *J. Ment. Defic. Res.* 31 (Pt. 1):73–9, 1987.

Hindler, CG, Norris, DL. A case of anorexia nervosa with Klinefelter's syndrome, *Br. J. Psychiatry* 149:659–60, 1986.

Bender, BG, Puck, MH, Salbenblatt, JA, Robinson, A. Dyslexia in 47,XXY boys identified at birth, *Behav. Genet.* 16(3):343–54, 1986.

Stein, MB, Siddiqui, AR. Acute paranoid disorder and Klinefelter's syndrome, *Can. J. Psychiatry* 31(5):434–5, 1986.

Singh, TH, Rajkowa, S. 49, XXXXY chromosome anomaly: An unusual variant of Klinefelter's syndrome, *Br. J. Psychiatry* 148:209–10, 1986.

Fryns, JP, Kleczkowska, A, Kubien, E, Van den Berghe, H. Cytogenetic findings in moderate and severe mental retardation: A study of an institutionalized population of 1991 patients, *Acta Paediatr. Scand. Suppl.* 1984;313:1–23, 1984.

Theilgaard, A. A psychological study of the personalities of XYY- and XXY-men, *Acta. Psychiatr. Scand. Suppl.* 315:1–133, 1984.

Cohen, FL, Durham, JD. Sex chromosome variations in school-age children, *J. Sch. Health* 55(3):99–102, 1985.

Cohen, FL, Durham, JD. Klinefelter syndrome, *J. Psychosoc. Nurs. Ment. Health Serv.* 23(1):19–25, 1985.

Fryns, JP. X-linked mental retardation, *Prog. Clin. Biol. Res.* 177:309–19, 1985.

Walzer, S. X chromosome abnormalities and cognitive development: Implications for understanding normal human development, *J. Child Psychol. Psychiatry* 26(2):177–84, 1985.

Garry, MB. Two cases of 48,XXYY: With discussion on the behaviour of prepubertal and postpubertal patients, *N. Z. Med. J.* 23;92(664):49–51, 1980.

Kunze, J. Neurological disorders in patients with chromosomal anomalies, *Neuropadiatrie* 11(3):203–49, 1980.

XYY Syndrome

Odetti, P, Del Nero, E, Bertora, G, Pizio, N, et al. XYY syndrome. A report of a juvenile case, *Minerva Endocrinol.* 13(1):13–5, 1988.

Benet, J, Martin, RH. Sperm chromosome complements in a 47,XYY man, *Hum. Genet.* 78(4):313–5, 1988.

Schiavi, RC, Theilgaard, A, Owen, DR, White, D. Sex chromosome anomalies, hormones, and sexuality, *Arch. Gen. Psychiatry* 45(1):19–24, 1988.

Cohen, FL, Durham, JD. Children with sex chromosome variations: Implications for pediatric nursing practice, *J. Pediatr. Nurs.* 1(1):12–23, 1986.

Kitsiou, S, Bartsocas, CS. Unusual association of XYY chromosomal constitution with colobomas of iris, myopia, increased lipoproteins, mental retardation and convulsions, *Ann. Genet.* (Paris) 29(4):264–5, 1986.

Theilgaard, A. A psychological study of the personalities of XYY- and XXY-men, *Acta. Psychiatr. Scand. Suppl.* 315:1–133, 1984.

Lake, CR, Baksh, HR, Wiedeking, C, Chernow, B, et al. Sympathetic nervous system function in XYY subjects, *Psychiatry Res.* 9(2):149–55, 1983.

Cohen, FL, Durham, JD. Sex chromosome variations in school-age children, *J. Sch. Health* 55(3):99–102, 1985.

Varrela, J, Alvesalo, L. Effects of the Y chromosome on quantitative growth: An anthropometric study of 47,XYY males, *Am. J. Phys. Anthropol.* 68(2):239–45, 1985.

Chandley, AC. Infertility and chromosome abnormality, *Oxf. Rev. Reprod. Biol.* 1984;6:1–46, 1984.

Gillberg, C, Winnergard, I, Wahlstrom, J. The sex chromosomes—One key to autism? An XYY case of infantile autism, *Appl. Res. Ment. Retard.* 5(3):353–60, 1984.

Bender, BG, Puck, MH, Salbenblatt, JA, Robinson, A. The development of four unselected 47,XYY boys, *Clin. Genet.* 25(5):435–45, 1984.

Schiavi, RC, Theilgaard, A, Owen, DR, White, D. Sex chromosome anomalies, hormones, and aggressivity, *Arch. Gen. Psychiatry* 41(1):93–9, 1984.

Theilgaard, A. Aggression and the XYY personality, *Int. J. Law Psychiatry* 6(3-4):413–21, 1983.

Mednick, SA, Finello, KM. Biological factors and crime: Implications for forensic psychiatry, *Int. J. Law Psychiatry* 6(1):1–15, 1983.

References

Baird, PA, Anderson, TW, Newcombe, HB, et al. Genetic disorders in children and young adults: A population study, *Am. J. Human Genet.* 42:677–693, 1988.

Brown, WT, Cohen, IL, Fisch, GS, Wolf-Shein, EG, Jenkins, EC. High dose folic acid treatment of fragile X males, *Am. J. Med. Genet.* 23:263–271, 1986.

Brown, WT, Jenkins, EC, Freidman, E, Brooks, J, Cohen, IL, Duncan, C, Hill, AL, Malik, MN, Morris, V, Wolf, E, Wisniewski, K, French, JH. Folic acid therapy in the fragile X syndrome, *Am. J. Med. Genet.* 17:289–297, 1984.

Brown, WT. The fragile X syndrome, *Neurol. Clin.* 7(1):107–21, 1989. Cartwright, GE, Diagnosis of treatable Wilson's disease, *New Engl. J. Med.* 298:1347–1350, 1978.

Comings, DE, Comings, BG. A controlled study of Tourette syndrome. I. Attention-deficit disorder, learning disorders, and school problems, *Am. J. Hum. Genet.* 41(5):701–41, 1987.

Cruikshank, WK. *Learning Disability in Home, School, and Community,* Syracuse University Press, Syracuse, NY, 1979.

281

Emery, AE, Rimoin, DL. *Principles and Practice of Medical Genetics*, Churchill Livingstone, New York, 1983.

Fisch, GS, Cohen, IL, Gross, AC, Jenkins, V, Jenkins, E, Brown, WT. Folic acid treatment of fragile X males: A further study, *Am. J. Med. Genet.*, 30:393-399, 1988.

Graham JM Jr, Bashir AS, Stark RE, Silbert A, Walzer S. Oral and written language abilities of XXY boys: Implications for anticipatory guidance. *Pediatrics* 81(6):795–806, 1988.

Gustavson, KH, Hagberg, B, Hagberg, C, Sars, K. Severe mental retardation in a Swedish county I. Epidemiology, gestational age, birth weight, and associated CNS handicaps in children born 1959–1970, *Acta Paediatrica* 66:373, 1977.

Gustavson, KH, Hagberg, B, Hagberg, C, Sars, K. Severe mental retardation in a Swedish county II. Etiological and pathologenetic aspects in children born 1959–1970, *Neuropadiatrica* 8:293-304, 1977.

Gastafson, K-H, Dahlbom, K, Holmgren, G, Blomquist, HK, Sanner, G. Effect of folic acid treatment in the fragile X syndrome, *Clin. Genet.* 27:463–467, 1985.

Jones, KL, *Smith's Recognizable Patterns of Human Malformation*, 4th ed., W.B. Saunders, Philadelphia, 1988.

Kanner, D. Autistic disturbances of affective contact, *Nerv. Child* 2:217-250, 1943.

Kanner, D. Emotional interference with emotional functioning, *Am. J. Ment. Dys.* 56:701–707, 1952.

Kaveggia, EG, Durkin, MV, Pendleton, E, Optitz JM. Diagnostic/genetic studies on 1224 patients with severe mental retardation. Proceedings of the 3rd Congress of the International Association for the Scientific Study of Mental Retardation. Polish Medical Publishers, Warsaw, 1975, pp 82–93.

Laxova, R, Ridler, MAC, Bowen-Bravery, M. An etiological survey of the severely retarded Hatfordshire children who were born between January 1, 1965 and December 31, 1967. *Am. J. Med. Genet.* 1:75-86, 1977.

McKusick, VA, *Mendelian Inheritance in Man*, 7th ed., Johns Hopkins University Press, Baltimore, 1986.

Meyen, EL, Public Law 94-142: Comments on the pediatricians' contribution from an educator, *Pediatrics*, 491–494, 1982.

Minshew, NJ, Payton JB. New perspectives in autism, Part I: The clinical spectrum of autism, *Curr. Probl. Pediatr.* 18(10):561–610, 1988.

Minshew, NJ, Payton, JB. New perspectives in autism, Part II: The differential diagnosis and neurobiology of autism. *Curr. Probl. Pediatr.* 18(11):613–94, 1988.

Moser, HW, Ramey, CT, Leonard CO, Mental retardation, 1982, in Emery AE, andRimoin DE (eds.) *Principles and Practice of Medical Genetics*, Churchill Livingston, New York, 1983, pp 352–366.

Nielsen, J, Pelsen, B. Follow-up 20 years later of 34 Klinefelter males with karyotype 47,XXY and 16 hypogonadal males with karyotype 46,XY. *Hum. Genet.* 77(2):188–92, 1987.

Ramey, CT, Finklestein, NW, Psychosocial mental retardation: A biological and social coalescence. In Begab, M, Haywood, C, Garber, H. (eds.) *Psychosocial Issues in Retarded Performance: Issues and Theories in Development*, University Park Press, Baltimore, 1981.

Sattler, J. *Assessment of Children*, 3rd ed., Jerome M. Sattler, San Diego, 1988.

Scriver, CR, Beaudet, AL, Sly, WS, Valle, D, *The Metabolic Basis of Inherited Disease*, 6th ed., McGraw-Hill, New York, 1989.

Shaywitz SE, Shaywitz, BA. Attention deficit disorder: Current perspectives. *Pediatr. Neurol.* 3(3):129-35, 1987.

Snyderman, M, Rothman, S. Survey of expert opinions on intelligence and aptitude testing, *Amer. Psychol.* 42:137-144, 1987.

Strom, CM, *Have a Healthy Baby*, Prentice-Hall, Englewood Cliffs, 1988.

Thompson, JS, Thompson, MW, *Genetics in Medicine*, 4th ed., W.B. Saunders Co, Philadelphia, 1986.

Tyler, E (ed.) *The Hyperactive Child, Clinics in Dev. Med. 97*, J.B. Lippincott, Philadelphia, 1986.

du Verglas, G, Banks, SR, Guyer, KE. Clinical effects of fenfluramine on children with autism: A review of the research. *J. Autism Dev. Disord.* 18(2):297–308, 1988.

Wright, GF. The pediatrician's role in Public Law 94–142, *Pediatrics in Rev.*, 4:191–197, 1982.

Index

285